THE GOOD GIRL RX

**Breaking Free from
Good Girl Syndrome**
to Heal Your Body,
Transform Your Relationships
and Uplevel Your Confidence

KATE BARTLEY, PT

©2025 by Kate Bartley

Published by hope*books
2217 Matthews Township Pkwy
Suite D302
Matthews, NC 28105
www.hopebooks.com

hope*books is a division of hope*media

Printed in the United States of America

All rights reserved. Without limiting the rights under copyrights reserved above, no part of this publication may be scanned, uploaded, reproduced, distributed, or transmitted in any form or by any means whatsoever without express prior written permission from both the author and publisher of this book—except in the case of brief quotations embodied in critical articles and reviews.

Thank you for supporting the author's rights.

First paperback edition.
Paperback ISBN: 979-8-89185-161-0
Hardcover ISBN: 979-8-89185-162-7
Ebook ISBN: 979-8-89185-163-4
Library of Congress Number 2025931416

All Scripture quotations, unless otherwise indicated, are taken from the Holy Bible, New International Version®, NIV®. Copyright ©1973, 1978, 1984, 2011 by Biblica, Inc.™ Used by permission of Zondervan. All rights reserved worldwide. www.zondervan.com The "NIV" and "New International Version" are trademarks registered in the United States Patent and Trademark Office by Biblica, Inc.™
Scripture quotations are from The ESV® Bible (The Holy Bible, English Standard Version®), © 2001 by Crossway, a publishing ministry of Good News Publishers. Used by permission. All rights reserved.
Scripture quotations marked MSG are taken from The Message, copyright © 1993, 2002, 2018 by Eugene H. Peterson. Used by permission of NavPress. All rights reserved. Represented by Tyndale House Publishers.

Scripture taken from the New King James Version®. Copyright © 1982 by Thomas Nelson. Used by permission. All rights reserved.

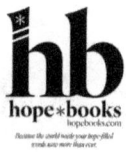

Table Of Contents

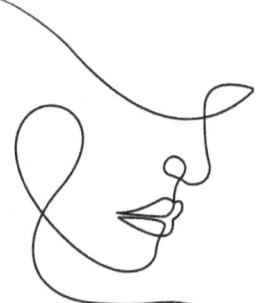

Prologue:
The "Good Girl's" Wake Up Call: My Body's Cry For Help 1

PART ONE:
THE GOOD GIRL WHO DENIED HERSELF 9

Chapter 1:
Defining Good Girl Syndrome 11

Chapter 2:
When Will My Life Begin? The Internal War and
Dreams Deferred 17

Chapter 3:
The Hidden Toll of the Good Girl 23

Chapter 4:
When the Good Girl Gets Sick 35

Chapter 5:
Learning to Be Good: The Hidden Cost of Praise
and Approval 45

Chapter 6:
The Weight of Good Intentions: Going Beyond Our Limits 53

PART TWO:
**THE GOOD GIRL WHO BEGAN TO UNDERSTAND
HER BODY** 63

Chapter 7:
When Normal Doesn't Feel Normal: Understanding and Healing the Body's Trauma Responses 65

Chapter 8:
Running for Peace: Escaping Discomfort Through the Flight Response 75

Chapter 9:
Unleashing Her Roar: Facing Conflict and Transforming Defensiveness into Healthy Aggression 89

Chapter 10:
Conditioned to Fawn: Unpacking Habits of Pleasing and Appeasing 103

Chapter 11:
Paralyzed by Fear: Understanding Her Freeze Response 117

Chapter 12:
From Repression to Expression: Feel to Heal 123

PART THREE:
THE GOOD GIRL WHO FACED HER BURIED FEARS 135

Chapter 13:
Hidden Stressors: Attachment Insecurity and Codependent Patterns 137

Chapter 14:
Unraveling Anxiety: Hypervigilance and Restoring a Sense of Security 147

Chapter 15:
Finding Freedom in Setting Boundaries 157

Chapter 16:
Breaking Free From Self Sabotage 167

PART FOUR:
THE GOOD GIRL WHO FOUND HER TRUE SELF 175

Chapter 17:
Lost and Found: Losing Yourself in Relationships 177

Chapter 18:
Getting Unshackled From Shame 187

Chapter 19:
Beyond Labels: Recognizing the Good in All of Us 195

Chapter 20:
Getting to Know and Embracing Her Shadow 209

Chapter 21:
Breaking the Rules: No More Supposed To's 223

Chapter 22:
Stepping Into Empowerment: Moving Beyond
Good Girl Syndrome 237

Chapter 23:
The Best You: The Good Girl Whose Story Helped Another 243

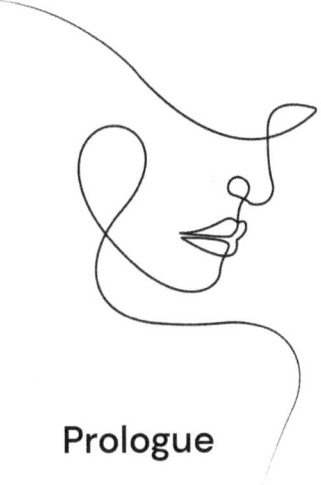

Prologue

The "Good Girl's" Wake Up Call: My Body's Cry For Help

"Most of us carry chronic stress for so long we no longer recognize the weight of it. That's why I call it a grace when our bodies rebel. It's God's way of saying, 'No more.'"
Rebekah Lyons[1]

I was never the type of person that got "stressed out." I was always the "laid back, go with the flow, nothing rocks my boat" girl, not someone that had panic attacks. When the ER doctor told me all my tests came back normal and the chest pain, shortness of breath, and shaking I'd just experienced were likely due to stress, it felt like he was discounting my experience and accusing me of crying wolf. I wanted to stand up from my chair like a defendant and shout, *That's not possible! I was sitting in a movie theater 'relaxing' when this happened!*

---

1   Lyons, Rebekah. *You Are Free: Be Who You Already Are.* Zondervan, 2017.

I was watching the newest Star Wars movie with my husband when I started feeling discomfort in my chest. I attributed it to heartburn and indigestion from the fried food I had for dinner and tried to ignore it, but it kept growing in intensity and affected my ability to relax. I finally excused myself to the bathroom, where I tried belching to relieve the pressure so I could go back and enjoy the movie. When I returned to my seat, however, my breathing became more and more labored, and my legs started tingling. I tried putting them up on the seat in front of me. I told myself I was fine and that it would go away if I ignored it, but it didn't. The educated part of me was scanning the sensations and comparing them to what I knew about circulation, while the part of me that just wanted to enjoy my date night kept saying, *We're fine. It's just indigestion.* But no matter how much I tried to calm myself, it just kept escalating until I finally turned to my husband and said, "I have to get out of here. I can't breathe." I now know my body was doing exactly what it was designed to do when it perceives a life threat: sounding an internal alarm and shouting, *Run! Get away! Do something!*

My husband followed me out to the parking lot and asked, "Do you want me to go get the truck, or can you make it?" I stood frozen in fear, gripping a nearby bench, torn between him leaving me alone and the stamina required to go with him. "I can't," I said. "I'll wait for you here," and as he ran, I prayed, *God, help me.*

Once in the truck, he continued asking me questions to determine the seriousness of what was happening. "Do you need to go to the hospital?" he asked.

"No," I answered without hesitation. I was fine. I could handle this. I just needed to go home and lie down and figure out how to get my body to relax. He started heading for the house, but instead of relaxing, a deep sense of dread and urgency filled me. *This isn't good. Something's not right. God, I don't want to die. What if I go home and there's no time to get back?*

With tears streaming down my face, I pushed through the embarrassment and forced a counter request, "I think I need to go to the hospital. Please take me there." I was mortified that I asked him to do that, like it was some kind of moral failure or weakness or something. My husband pulled up to the revolving door just outside the ER, and someone came out with a wheelchair. They helped me into it as he parked. I felt so stupid for needing it and wanted to walk, but my body was shaking violently by that time. As my husband filled out the paperwork for me, I planted both hands on my legs, willing them to stop their pendulations, thinking, *What is wrong with me? Why am I shaking like this?*

I was wheeled past the waiting room into a private space where they pulled a white curtain around me, placed electrodes on my chest, and checked my heart rhythm. Once satisfied that I was stable, we were directed back to the crowded room with everyone else they'd triaged as "good to wait." It felt like being abandoned, like what I was experiencing didn't warrant care and attention, like they assumed I was capable of handling it on my own, which was bumping up against the narrative I had to overcome to get myself there. There was no way in hell I'd have come to the ER asking for help if there wasn't something seriously wrong. I was a medical professional myself! I know the difference between stress and a serious problem! I'd had annual CPR training on the warning signs of a heart attack, and I'd just experienced all of them. I'd done what I was supposed to and gone to the hospital; I knew better than to ignore them. But here I sat with no other explanation offered. I couldn't wrap my head around the idea that the sense of dread I'd just experienced could have been stress-induced. I didn't share their confidence. I didn't feel safe enough to be left there. I still couldn't breathe.

I slid back in the chair and shifted my body over and over again, trying desperately to find some kind of relief. I was still shaking when a young girl came to escort me to radiology for a chest x-ray. Once inside, she directed me to stand up. My eyes shouted, *Do you not see me? I can't even sit up in this chair right now, and you want me to stand?* My eyes must have gotten the message across, as she finally reached down to offer me assistance. Her help, while appreciated, felt more like an impatient mother reaching down to tie her child's shoe so they could get out the door. Once the x-rays were captured, she wheeled me right back out, never once asking if I was okay. I felt like a task she was checking off on her list of things to do.

After over an hour, someone finally came out and gave us a report: "All your tests look okay, but we want you to stick around and have blood drawn one more time." I looked at my husband and declared, "Get me out of here. I want to go home."

I don't know if I was humiliated, mad, or impatient—maybe all three—but I didn't care what they recommended at that point. I was done waiting for them to provide the reassurance and comfort my body needed. I could take it from there. I messaged my doctor and scheduled an appointment to follow up with him the next morning.

My doctor was caring enough to try to help me sort through what might have happened and run any additional tests. We decided to check my thyroid levels to see if that might be related to my symptoms. However, without any further explanation, I was left with the unsettling experience unresolved and without any guidance on how to prevent it from happening again. It felt like being robbed and never catching the burglar. It's hard to sleep at night when you don't know where the enemy is... or if they intend to come back.

Before I was diagnosed with Papillary Thyroid Cancer, I never worried about my health. I had a habit of ignoring my symptoms and pushing through pain. If I woke up sick, I drugged myself and kept going unless my body forced me horizontal through a stomach virus or dizziness. I was a mom, a physical therapist, and a children's ministry leader. I didn't have time to be sick. People needed me. Even with my experience in healthcare, I was unaware that the events occurring in my life and the struggles within my soul over the past few months could impact my neurobiology and my ability to fend off illness. I didn't understand how stress, unresolved trauma, and my learned attachment and survival habits were contributing to my distress and dis-ease.

What I experienced in that ER was more than just a health scare—it was a wake-up call that shattered my belief that I was "fine" and forced me to confront a reality I had long ignored. I realized my body had been trying to speak to me for years, but I hadn't been listening. This experience revealed the connection between the stress I denied and the "Good Girl" conditioning that had shaped my life. As I delved deeper, I discovered I was not alone. Women everywhere face the same invisible chains that keep them from thriving, struggling under the weight of expectations, and losing touch with their own needs. My story is just one example of how "Good Girl" conditioning can lead to unexpected health crises.

I wrote this book to shed light on unhealthy patterns, unravel their complexities, and offer a path to transformation and healing. Unlearning these patterns was the key to restoring my own health when nothing in the traditional medical model was working. Each chapter will end with a section called "Good Girl Rx,"—a reflective tool designed to help you untangle these patterns in your own life. These reflections aren't just about recognizing the traps that may be hindering your well-being, but uncovering a path to freedom. Take time to sit with these questions and let them guide you toward clarity, self-compassion, and growth.

I believe, along with many renowned physicians and healers– including Jesus himself–that these shifts in my soul restored life to my body. We're discovering the scientific basis of what we've long known but forgotten: the deep connection between our spiritual and physical bodies. This is a Biblical approach, and one that Jesus modeled. He never addressed the body without addressing underlying issues in the context of people's lives. He knew healing was a byproduct of wholeness and always used this inside-out approach.

Through self-examination, insight, and listening to our bodies, we can embark on the transformational journey that Jesus invites us into: one of restoration and renewal. We must come back home to the truth and goodness of who we inherently are, shedding the "Good Girl" persona that has become too heavy for us to wear. It's an invitation to reclaim our birthright to need and receive, find our voices, trust our bodies' innate wisdom, and live in alignment with God's heart for us. It's a prescription for our healing.

Over the past 10 years, I've studied everything from women's hormones, habit psychology, attachment patterns, neuroplastic pain, nervous system regulation, somatic experiencing, the psychology of the soul, the biology of trauma, and transformational coaching. However, my most profound learning came from the laboratory of life—through my experiences and the stories of the women I've coached. I have the honor of providing a safe, supportive space that I needed but couldn't find for other nurturing, service-driven women whose bodies, like mine, express a cry for help they struggle to articulate. I love empowering them to uncover the source of their stress and symptoms so that they, too, can feel safe and at ease in their bodies again. I love guiding them out of their heads—where they're trying to figure out what's wrong with them—and into their bodies and souls, where they can reconnect with their gut wisdom, unmet needs, and deepest desires.

My reason for writing is simple: too many women are suffering and way too many are dying before ever getting to become grandmothers. My hope is that through my story, and the stories of the many women I've had the honor of helping, you will find clarity and actionable steps to start embodying your healthiest self and begin enjoying a lighter, more carefree way of being.

I pray that as you read, you'll start finding the courage to say "no" to what no longer serves you and discover the "yes" that enlivens you. My own "yes" was writing, and it brings me back to life every time I allow myself the freedom of expression. Writing this book is my way of embodying these healing principles, overcoming my insecurities, breaking free from the fear of judgment, and releasing the truths and stories I've been holding within me. I'm not writing from a place of arrival but as a fellow sojourner. This book is my hand reaching back to you. I invite you to take it and then reach out and grasp the hands of the women around you who need this too. Let's break free from "good girl" conditioning together and reclaim a life of authenticity, health, and unadulterated joy. This book is not just about identifying harmful patterns—it's about breaking free from them. Through self-compassion, recognition, and courage, we can become active agents of our healing, powerful advocates for our well-being, and co-creators of our lives.

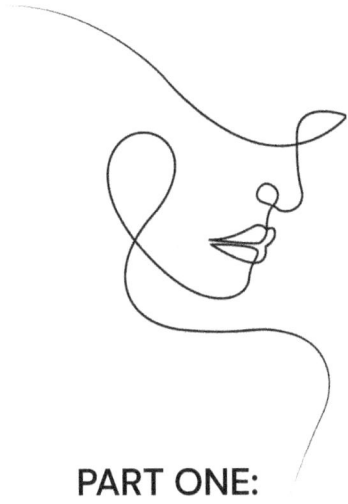

PART ONE:

THE GOOD GIRL WHO DENIED HERSELF

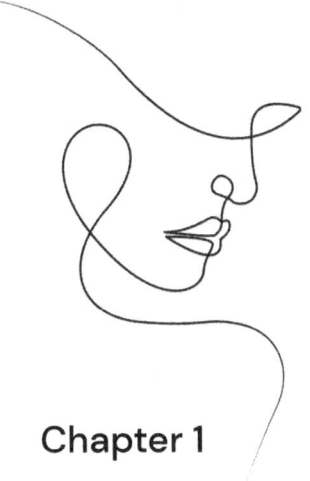

Chapter 1

Defining Good Girl Syndrome

"Until you make the unconscious conscious, it will direct your life and you will call it fate."
Carl Jung[2]

One morning, while visiting my daughter and son-in-law, I woke up to the sound of strong, declarative "no's" coming from my granddaughter's bedroom. I smiled and got curious about what she was refusing. After a few minutes, it became clear there was no one in her room trying to force her to get dressed, have her diaper changed, or brush her hair. She was simply articulating her desires. *No, I don't want to look at this book. No, not this one either. Ah, this is the one I want.* No one was invading her boundaries or getting in her space. She was just practicing her birthright to decide her preferences, and there was nothing

---

2   While this is not a direct quote from Jung, it is a summation of his thoughts as presented in: Jung, C.G. *Aion: Researches into the Phenomenology of the Self.* Translated by R.F.C. Hull, Princeton University Press, 1951.

hindering her from stating them. She hadn't yet learned that expressing what you want or don't want is not always acceptable.

This is the innocence of childhood: the pure expression of our desires without feeling shame for wanting, the fear of others' reactions, or being flooded with guilt over how our choices might affect them. There's nothing holding us back. This is what we need to restore if we are ever going to walk in wellness and become empowered women.

So why do so many women end up struggling with this? What causes us to silence our voices, feel selfish for expressing our desires, or ask for what we need? At some point, a little girl starts learning that her honest expression isn't always safe.

She learns that:

- Voicing her preferences can cause others to pull away or become upset with her.
- Her restraint and obedience gets praised and rewarded.
- Demanding less eases the stress on her caregivers.
- Being quiet and reserved is more socially acceptable.

These lessons foster a pattern of self-suppression, where the need for attachment overrides authenticity and instinctual responses. Over time, these behaviors become unconscious habits, shaping our self-perception, worldview, and relationships—including our relationship with God. Sadly, they can also hinder women from achieving their deepest desires and experiencing His heart for them. This is how the "Good Girl Syndrome" is formed, with profound and lasting effects on a woman's health and well-being.

What is "Good Girl Syndrome?"

"Good Girl Syndrome" is a set of learned behaviors and coping mechanisms many women unwittingly adapt that lead them to prioritize others' needs over their own, trapping them in childhood survival strategies that sabotage their personal well-being. These behaviors are often rooted in the belief that being good equates to selflessness and that self-suppression is necessary to earn love and acceptance. While prioritizing others can be a beautiful expression of love and care, it becomes harmful when it shifts from wholehearted giving to chronic self-abandonment. When serving others is driven by fear, guilt, or a need for approval, it can lead to overwhelm, anxiety, depression, mind-body syndromes, and even serious health conditions. If you constantly push yourself beyond your energetic capacity, prioritize others' needs over your own, feel guilty taking time for yourself, or rely on illness to give you permission to rest, you may be grappling with these deeply ingrained patterns.

In my work as a Mind Body Practitioner and Life Empowerment Coach, I've found this pattern to be the key barrier that keeps my clients from taking the action steps they know they need for their health and well-being. There is often so much guilt and shame entangling them and blocking them from moving forward. When we've been taught to be selfless, prioritizing our own needs doesn't feel doable. "Goodness," while often seen as virtuous, can perpetuate a cycle of stress and exhaustion when we forget to include ourselves on the list of people to be good too.

My intention isn't to pathologize this common and often necessary early conditioning but to highlight how these patterns, if left unchanged, can trap us in harmful habits that undermine our health. It's not about blaming anyone but understanding how these behaviors develop and impact our lives. Many women find themselves ensnared in this web of conditioning, struggling to say "no" and suppressing their needs and feelings. Our bodies often step in to set boundaries for us through chronic pain and stress-related illnesses when the risk of articulating our boundaries feels too great. The first step to breaking free from these traps is to reconnect with the part of yourself that was never meant to carry these burdens in the first place.

I invite you to reflect on the purity of expression my granddaughter enjoyed in her crib, unburdened by shame, fear, or guilt when articulating her needs and desires. Can you feel the safety of that? Now imagine this for all the babies in the world. Picture a hillside stretched before you, covered with thousands of little blankets, each cradling an innocent baby girl—girls of all nationalities and sizes. Walk gently between them, gazing into their tiny souls, and ask yourself: which one doesn't have the right to express herself? Which one doesn't deserve to reach for the wildflowers, crawl, explore, and cry out to be held when she is afraid? None of them deserve to be taught that their desires are wrong or that their needs are a burden. And neither do you. If you found yourself believing that one baby somehow didn't deserve it, consider this: just because we feel something doesn't make it true. What we feel as right or wrong, good or bad, has more to do with our programming and early experiences. The good news is that we can reclaim this innocence, the birthright to express ourselves and make life-giving choices without feeling guilty for doing so.

GOOD GIRL RX: Awaken To Create Transformation

Everything starts with awareness. We can't change what we're not conscious of. Start by getting a baseline of where you are now so you can reflect back later and see just how far you've come!

Good Girl Syndrome Self-Reflection Quiz

For each statement, please answer "Yes" or "No."
1. **Difficulty Saying "NO":** Do you find it challenging to say "NO" to requests, even when it inconveniences you?
2. **Taking on Others' Responsibilities:** Do you often take on the responsibility for meeting the needs of others, even when you're already stretched too thin?
3. **Emotional Suppression:** Do you suppress, internalize, or hide your emotions from others?

4. **Self-Sufficiency/Comfort in Independence:** Growing up, did you handle your problems independently without seeking much support or attention? Was it easier to do it yourself than to trust or depend on your primary caregiver? As an adult, do you feel more comfortable when you can take care of things on your own without relying on others?
5. **Fear of Upsetting Others:** Do you tend to avoid expressing your needs or desires because you are afraid it might upset or inconvenience someone else?
6. **Prioritizing Others' Comfort:** Do you frequently prioritize protecting others from pain or suffering while sacrificing your own comfort and discounting your needs or feelings?
7. **Rewarded for being Good:** As a child, did you receive praise or attention primarily when you were being helpful, well-behaved, or doing something good? Do you still feel the need for others' validation before taking action as an adult?
8. **Feeling Unseen or Misunderstood:** Do you often feel unseen, unheard, or misunderstood?
9. **Early Childhood Trauma:** Did you experience any form of childhood trauma like ongoing criticism, emotional or physical abuse or neglect, or a home environment filled with fear, anxiety, or insecurity? Do you still feel the effects of these experiences?
10. **Struggling with Self-Value:** Do you struggle to value yourself, express your feelings, or assert your boundaries when they are being violated?

This self-reflection quiz is just a starting point. Your answers are simply insights into the areas calling for attention, trailheads for transformation.

Take a moment to record your insights below. What areas are calling for attention and healing?

*To explore these patterns further and identify the specific traps affecting your well-being, visit https://katebartley.com for a more in-depth guide that will lead you through next steps toward freedom and healing.

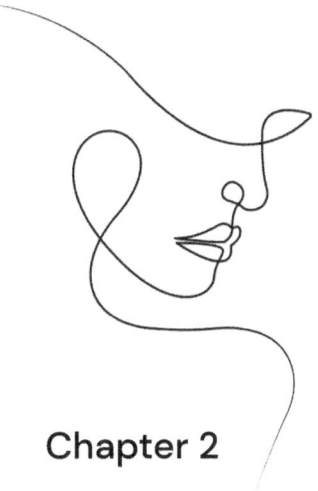

Chapter 2

When Will My Life Begin? The Internal War and Dreams Deferred

"It is for freedom that Christ has set us free. Stand firm, then, and do not let yourselves be burdened again by a yoke of slavery."
Galatians 5:1

The song "When Will My Life Begin" came on as I was finishing my morning run one day. The memory of a scene from the movie Tangled, Rapunzel spinning in circles in the grass, running through the breeze with arms outstretched in reckless abandon, made me smile. This is what breaking free from "Good Girl" conditioning looks and feels like.

There's another scene that highlights the internal war Rapunzel feels as she fights to break free. One moment, she's giddy with joy, spinning in freedom, and the next, she's chiding herself for wrecking her mother, calling herself a despicable daughter. It makes me laugh, but when you're caught in that stronghold, it's not so funny, is it?

Flynn Rider, depicted as the bad boy, notices her conflict and works to ease her conscience: "This is part of growing up. A little rebellion, a little adventure, that's good. Healthy, even." You can hear the self-doubt in her voice as she replies, "You think?" To which he asserts, "I know."[3] This confidence is what we have to reclaim if we're going to become our healthiest selves. Maybe you are asking the questions Rapunzel and many other women have wondered: *When will my life begin? When can I follow my heart's desire and do the thing that makes my soul sing?*

Maybe your soul is crying out for freedom in the same way mine was several years ago. Like Flynn Rider, I know shaking loose these strongholds is the pathway to growth and transformation. It's this restoration of deep security within our soul that activates the flow of health in our bodies and floods our minds with peace.

The War Within: My Breaking Point

Eight years ago, I stood in my kitchen with that war raging within me. Tears streamed down my face as I tried desperately to articulate to my husband what was going on internally.

We had just come home from seeing the movie *La La Land*, and a particular scene featuring the main actress sitting by an open window lost in her writing, following her dreams, deeply affected me. The part of me that longed for permission to do the same was overcome with grief that I'd never be given the chance, believing it wasn't possible and that it wasn't *God's will* for me.

I sat there trying to cover the flood of emotions with my hands, creating walls to hide the tears, willing myself to get it together, telling myself how crazy I was for falling apart in a musical rom-com. I thought, geez, what must my husband think? He watched this cheesy movie just for me, and this was how I show appreciation? I felt bad for not displaying gratitude for the

---

3   *Tangled*, directed by Nathan Greno and Byron Howard (Walt Disney Pictures, 2010), 00:33:06.

movie he selflessly chose to watch with me. I'd always been told to be grateful for the gifts I'd received and let others know how thankful I was. I guess that was the same reason I was chiding myself for my discontentment.

My husband kept asking, "What's wrong?" There was no hiding it anymore. The storm raging inside of me was seething out.

Have you ever felt completely stumped when someone asks you that? The words were frozen in my throat. It took everything in me to find my voice in that moment and admit my secret desires: "I want to write. I need to write," to which my husband replied, "Then do. What's stopping you?"

Here's what was stopping me: shame so thick you could cut it with a knife. With it came my fierce inner critic using guilt to put me back in line.

My inner monologue sounded something like this: *How stupid, Kate. What are you doing? How can you ask for something so self-centered? Your family needs you out there working, not hiding away behind a computer. You did this once before, remember? You weren't any good at it. No one was interested in what you had to say. If God wanted you to write, people would have been drawn to it. You're going to look like those American Idol contestants who think they can sing and then humiliate themselves instead. They think they are called to something but are deluding themselves. You need to be using your time doing something productive to help your family, and writing is not going to contribute anything to them.*

These voices from the past were my wall of Jericho, standing high around my heart, trying to keep me safe but keeping me contained. Letting him see my secret desires felt really scary. *What if he didn't validate them or show support? What if my need took away from his? What if my "dream" created a financial burden, or worse, what if he didn't believe in me?* And on the flip side, *what if he did support me?* Then I'd have nothing holding me back, and that's even scarier! I might have to take a step of courage! *But what If I didn't have what it takes to succeed?* No wonder I was trying to push all those emotions down!

That moment of radical honest expression was my act of bravery—my escape. Giving a voice to my secret desire broke the chains that were holding me captive. Taking that courageous step to express my intuitive needs was the catalyst that restored my health after a season of chronic symptoms and illness.

Maybe you're feeling the turmoil of being entangled by the same voices. Maybe, like Rapunzel, you have been trained to suppress your intuition, second-guess yourself, and trust that others know what's best for you, but there is a little girl inside you losing hope of ever being given permission to follow the lights outside her window. Like you, I have strong feelings of shame and guilt that act like guards. They try to keep me from going outside "God's" best for me. They warn me, saying, *Be careful. It isn't safe to go that way.* Do you hear the fear in that? The insecurity?

I stand with Flynn and say to you: Breaking free from that voice of shame is the healthiest thing you can do! It's a necessary step of growth. Left unchecked, it will keep you stuck, steal your joy, and cause you to miss the very thing God created for you to enjoy: abundant life.

When we constrain ourselves in order to stay safe, we block the very thing we're trying to protect and sabotage the thing we most desire: the freedom to live fully—to spin, roll in the grass, and have so much joy we laugh out loud. To climb trees, get dirty, and explore whatever our nose is drawn to along the way. Life is meant to be lived, not limited. One leads to health in the body, the other to inflammation and dis-ease.

GOOD GIRL RX: Embrace the Freedom to Follow Your Dreams

While the ER wake-up call revealed the physical toll of "Good Girl" conditioning, it only scratched the surface. The real battle lay within—a constant struggle between my deepest desires and the guilt and self-doubt that plagued me. Perhaps you've felt that inner conflict too—the pull between wanting to live fully and the fear that whispers, *Don't go that way. It's not safe.*

Breaking free begins with acknowledging this inner battle. As you reflect on this chapter, take a moment to consider the ways you might still be holding yourself back and how your life and health might change if you allowed yourself the freedom to pursue what God is inviting you into.

Reflection Questions:

1. What dream or longing has God placed in your heart that you haven't yet pursued? What's been holding you back? What's one small action you can take today to allow yourself to start exploring it?
2. What belief or fear might you need to let go of to take that first brave step?

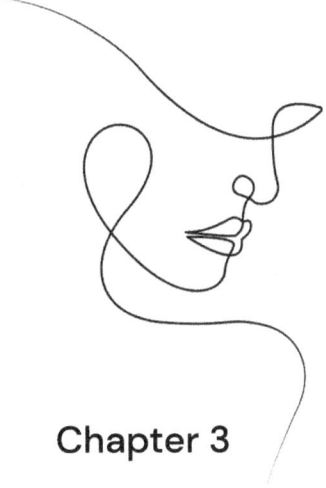

Chapter 3

The Hidden Toll of the Good Girl

"The compulsive and automatic concern for the needs of others while ignoring your own is a major risk factor for chronic illness"
Gabor Mate, M.D.[4]

I recently watched a documentary about the sexual and psychological abuse that took place within the US gymnastics culture, and my jaw dropped as I listened to the testimonials of the girls I grew up idolizing.

The most impactful statement was this:

> "We were taught to ignore our own feelings, so when medical professionals told us something was standard treatment, we doubted our instincts and trusted them. When we felt pain in our knees or exhaustion, we were told it was nothing.

---

4   Maté, Gabor. *When the Body Says No: The Cost of Hidden Stress*. Vintage Canada, 2004. Quote is a summation of the ideas presented within the book.

This habit of disregarding our own feelings and experiences made us vulnerable to mistreatment. We were praised for ignoring our discomfort and obeying authority figures." (*Athlete A 00:45:30*).

We see these exceptional young girls, sometimes only thirteen or fourteen, doing things with such precision and ease that awe and inspire us, making us want to be like them. I remember admiring their discipline, work ethic, commitment, and determination, the way their bodies were sculpted and shaped, and the way they held back tears when they fell and got right back up again. I never realized the "training" that went into that went far beyond physical conditioning.

At the last Olympic Games, Simone Biles, the most decorated gymnast of all time, who was expected to take home the gold, was called "weak" for listening to her intuition and pulling herself out of the competition to honor her needs and heed her body's danger signals. When she returned home, she received backlash from the American Public: "She should have pushed through." That is, after all, what we've been conditioned to value: strong, selfless women who deny their pain and are willing to suffer for the benefit of others. We highlight it in their obituaries.

No wonder we suffer in silence. No wonder we break down. We live in a culture of suck it up and sacrifice yourself, and our churches reinforce it. This is the calling card of the "Good Girl," and I am a recovering one myself. I know firsthand the toll it can take on our health.

Exhaustion and Depletion: The Danger of Selfless Service

I'd been serving as a Children's Ministry Director at a Church Plant for seven years when my body gave me an out through Thyroid Cancer.

At the onset of our journey, when my husband shared the vision God had laid on his heart to come alongside our friends and plant a church, shedding tears as he spoke, my gut had reservations, but how could I say no? I loved seeing his passion, and I'd been praying for years for God to show us how we could serve Him side by side. I'd been taught that my purpose as a wife was to be his helpmate, to encourage and support him to use his gifts in leadership. Here was my opportunity! I saw it as a chance to feel closer and find unity in a shared purpose, so I set aside my own reservations.

This was the mindset I carried into the church plant, one that had been ingrained into me from an early age and deepened with other things my brain absorbed as a good Christian girl. There were Scripture passages and messages hidden in my heart so "I might not sin against Him," but they weren't just written on my heart—they were etched into my brain and woven into my nervous system.

Joy = Jesus first, then others, and finally, yourself.
Put others first. Put yourself last.
Your heart is deceitful and cannot be trusted.
God made me in order to meet my husband's need for companionship. My purpose is to help him. Being a helpmate is an honor!

These were the narratives that had shaped me.

I know what you're thinking, *But Kate, you're taking these out of context!* Yes, I am. That's the point. Our unconscious mind does this all the time. It's called confirmation bias. It reads and hears everything through the lens of our early experiences, so every time these narratives are preached, taught, or underlined in a Bible Study, those neurological wires become stronger. *What fires together, wires together.* It's basic neuroscience working at its finest. It doesn't matter how much you tell me God loves me and cares for me or that Jesus gave his own life to die for me; my subconscious is holding a different story—stories that say-

I'm less important.
God values others more than me.
The only way to feel close to Him is to please Him.

This is exactly what I did for seven years at our church plant. I could count on one hand the number of times I attended service with other adults in a posture where I could receive my own nourishment. What started as excitement about getting to be a part of something bigger than myself left me feeling more isolated and alone than I'd ever been. I felt disconnected from what everyone else was experiencing, never getting to be involved or even witness it. I was in the back, caring for the needs of the kids and making sure their parents could experience God's love for them. *Less of me, more of Him. Less of me, more for them...*

It finally took a toll on me, and I found myself crying myself to sleep on Saturday nights, shouting at God and telling Him I was done. *I'm not doing this anymore! This is not healthy! I am not getting up and going in the morning!*

Can you hear the authentic "no's" of the little one within me voicing her preferences in the safety of her bedroom? Only, this went beyond preference. I was exercising my right to set a boundary in a place where it didn't feel so risky, where freedom of expression felt safe. I'd lay there thinking, *Why doesn't anyone see me? Why aren't they concerned about me like I would be for them? I would never let someone go week after week for seven years without being nurtured and fed. I would be checking in with them and asking if they were okay. Why don't they care that I'm overextended, unpaid, and doing more than my share? Can they not see that I'm clocking more hours than the pastor is? And why are we paying someone outside the church to come in and play music for an hour, but what*

I'm doing—which, by the way, is allowing them all to gather without distraction—is an unpaid, volunteer position? You might say, *But Kate, you were a grown-up, perfectly capable of speaking up for yourself, saying no, and telling them what needed to be different.* Well, it's like the gymnasts in the documentary I watched; I'd been conditioned not to. When I did mention I was struggling, I was encouraged to try lifting my eyes off my own problems and focus on someone else with the added projection. *"That always helps me!"* I knew in the depths of my soul that when I was given that advice, it wasn't right for me. Everything in me screamed, *No! That's the last thing I need right now!*

In my bed that night, that "no" raged within me, demanding to be heard, even if God and I were the only ones privy to it. On the other side of my anger, buried sadness found space to release, and I felt a shift in my body as my soul let it all out, allowing me to settle into sleep—just like I often did as a "good" baby, without "needing" anyone to comfort me. I made sure my screams were muffled by my pillow or the walls of my closet, far from anyone's ears, leaving my husband and everyone else completely unaware of how much I was silently struggling.

The next morning, I'd wake up knowing that *not going* wasn't an option. I couldn't bear what that might do to my family. I'd be pulling them down with me, and that went against my core values. *Better a millstone be tied around my neck and I be cast into the sea to drown than to cause my own husband and children to stumble."*[5] No, I had to get up, be strong, find a way to say yes to my assignment and worship where God had called me. So I did, again and again and again.

To be honest, I really did realign my heart before I stood on that stage and taught those kids. I never carried that resentment with me or spoke inauthentically. This "Good Girl" was not in the

---

5   "It would be better for him if a millstone were hung around his neck and he were cast into the sea than that he should cause one of these little ones to sin." Luke 17:2, ESV

habit of pretending. Honesty was a core value, too; well, with the exception of what I didn't say, I guess. I was never inauthentic with God, and He met me there in my screams and surrender and lifted me each and every time. The next week, the same shout from my soul would remind me this was not healthy for me to continue with.

But another part of me would recite Galatians 6:9, "Don't become weary in doing good, for at the proper time you will reap a harvest if you do not give up." and the part that was raising a white flag begging to be noticed would be silenced like a lamb. I mean, that is what Jesus would do, right? I was taught to follow Him into self-sacrifice, so I did, week in and week out, believing it was right. Well, at least one part of me did. I guess I assumed the crying, angry, weary parts were just my "flesh" lashing out. Those were the parts I was supposed to deny, right? Matthew 16:24-25 (NKJV) echoed in my ear, "If anyone desires to come after Me, let him deny himself, and take up his cross, and follow Me." So I followed. I obeyed. I ignored the cries of my soul and put on my big girl pants week after week.

It wasn't this way the whole time. I loved the planning, searching for curriculum, and even writing and creating my own at times. I loved using my child development experience to engage the kids and imprint the truth that God cared about more than their obedience, that He longed for their joy and pleasure, too. I loved building a team and seeing women new to the church learn to understand God in a whole new way as they served and studied the Bible passage each week. I loved teaching and speaking and seeing the smiles on their faces and the lightbulbs in their eyes.

It made sense for me to say yes to directing and developing the program; I mean, I was the one with the child development background, and we needed someone to do it. The only problem was that it wasn't the vision God had given me when I said "yes" to being a part of the launch team. My heart had gotten excited about *collaborating* with the team, gathering and brainstorming and building this together, and praying with and for each other. I saw the potential to be a part of creating an atmosphere of belonging and to experience that myself. Once we launched the church, the demands quickly became overwhelming, and my own needs were pushed aside. Each of us focused on ensuring that everything was done with excellence so that the people God sent would have their needs met. That would become the common denominator in my life when it came to being stretched too thin.

I actually prided myself on my ability to protect margin in my life–for the most part. I'd stepped back from working full time after my first child was born and always took a daily nap when my kids did. I wasn't usually in the habit of abandoning my needs. I knew how to care for others and have plenty of time for myself. I made self-care a priority because I wanted to be rested and filled up, so I had something left for my husband in the evening. I knew how important it was to guard our relationship, and that meant guarding myself. I knew if my needs were met and my soul was full, I could say yes to doing something he preferred, like watching a John Wayne episode. I could choose sacrifice in a genuine altruistic way.

What I learned, however, is this all goes out the window when the needs around me start to rise, and I sense there's no one else available to meet them without being burdened by them. This is exactly what happened in the church.

I tried to step back multiple times. My intention was to get a team of people on a rotating schedule, including teaching leaders, and step back so the program could run itself and I could go into the service. The problem was we were a small church, a transition point for people who were trying to plug back in. Once they did, they often ended up leaving to find something bigger. Just when I thought I was going to be able to attend the service, a hole would develop, and I would step in to prevent someone else who needed a break from having to fill it.

I hated seeing people not having their needs met. I didn't mind asking them to serve, but I was never going to let them do too much. I knew it wasn't healthy for them. Putting someone else in a toxic position was a big fat no for me, so I just kept swimming in the green stuff myself.

I tried pleading with my husband a few times, demanding a reason for why he felt compelled to stay. His answer was always, "Until God closes this door or opens another one, this is where He has called us to stay."

"But why?" I asked. "Why do you feel called to this? I mean, how do you know this is where God wants us? How in the world could it be His will for us to stay in something that's not healthy for me?" Despite my questioning, his commitment remained steadfast. He truly believed we should stay until God showed us otherwise. I don't blame him for that. I was taught the same thing.

My husband did encourage me to advocate for myself. He was all for me bringing the kids into the service when there wasn't enough help or shifting the responsibility back onto the parents. We tried having the kids start in the service and worship with the parents so at least I got to be a part of that, which helped, but it's not easy to worship when you're noticing all the distracted and frustrated parents.

In hindsight, I can see more options. Why didn't I go to other churches, speak at Sunday school classes, or find more volunteers? Why didn't we share the vision and provide opportunities for more people to be involved? Likely because we'd all experienced the sting of rejection too many times before. It was easier to do it ourselves than to risk the pain of being told "no." It doesn't matter how much we know there are other possibilities if our bodies sense a risk. I can't say for certain, but I imagine I wasn't alone in feeling depleted.

The Sunday School answer to that is "Cast your cares upon me," or to "Let go and let God, " or "In our weakness, He is strong." Basically, stop trying to do it with your own strength. These are all beautiful truths, but we have this habit of assuming it's pride that keeps us from stepping back when usually it's fear. That fear is not something we can just pray away. It's embedded in our nervous systems.

This is why we get on our knees, try to release something, and five minutes later, we've picked it back up again. If our body senses a danger or threat, our subconscious is going to take over and activate our survival habits. When I perceived others might suffer if my needs were met, it felt too threatening to express that or ask for my own needs to be met. I knew rationally that both my needs and others' needs could coexist, but that didn't make it feel any safer.

Acknowledging the Toll of Self-Sacrifice

Reflecting on the situation now, I realize it wasn't the work that took a toll on me but the loneliness and isolation I felt. We can endure so much when we lean on each other. That's the beauty of how we're designed—our stress response is calmed through connection and co-regulation with others. This is the gift of a healthy community—a body of people holding and supporting one another. In my faith, it's what the body of Christ is meant to be: each person playing a part so no one carries the burden alone. But I didn't feel held together. I felt isolated and alone.

We are all born with the right to need—to express our desires for connection, care, and support. But somewhere along the way, I learned to suppress that right, burying my needs so deeply that even I couldn't recognize them clearly. I wanted help but didn't know how to ask for it. I thought my struggles were obvious—like I was waving a white flag—but it was invisible.

Many "Good Girls" become so aware of others' facial expressions, tone of voice, and what's going on in their environment that if they perceive it's not safe to ask for what they need, they will shut down, go mum, or flee. That's what kept happening to me. We become so highly attuned to others to make sure what we're asking for is okay–that it isn't going to put anyone out or be perceived as rude or selfish. If we get the impression that might happen, our inner coach blows the whistle to punt. We learn when it's safe to speak up and when to swallow our words. The more important the "game" is, the less risk we're willing to take. I guess the church was just a place where it felt necessary to play it safe.

I was afraid of speaking up and standing up for my needs for rest, to step back and take a break, and I let others' expectations of themselves be projected onto me. No one else was expressing their needs, either. I didn't have anyone over me that was providing accountability or a healthy model. I was *trying really hard* to rely on God. I was in my Bible, diving deep into intimacy with Him, wrestling with Him, delighting in Him. He was, after all, the only one I could be radically honest with. He was my friend in the loneliness and the only thing sustaining me... at least until I started getting resentful that He wasn't rescuing me.

I don't think the problem was a lack of reliance on God but a lack of trust in people. I didn't feel secure enough in articulating my needs to others. I didn't want to be selfish or burden them. I knew God could handle my needs, anger, and tears, but I wasn't so sure they could.

This is an attachment trauma response, one many "Good Girls" have. It's what compels us to get into helping professions. We see people's needs because they're the very ones we long to have met ourselves. When we can't express our needs, it often takes something "valid" to give us permission to step back. It took a serious health issue and the church's financial struggles to give me a way out. While others prayed for resources to stay afloat, I silently hoped for relief. When our church merged with another congregation, it felt like my escape—a chance to step away from the endless demands and expectations. For the first time in years, I sat in church without the weight of responsibility.

Just weeks later, my doctor found the enlarged thyroid nodule—it was as if my body, in its wisdom, knew I needed a valid reason.

GOOD GIRL RX: Identify the Invisible Snares

My prayer has always been, *"God, don't ever let me be unaware."* I knew I couldn't change what I couldn't see. It's hard to avoid a snare in the path when it's covered by leaves. When we take the time to grow in understanding of what's been entangling us, we can open the door to greater choice and possibility.

Reflection Questions:

1. While reading this chapter, did you notice the traps that led to my inevitable burnout while serving at the church? Take a moment to name them.
2. Which of these traps have you fallen into in your own life?
3. How have these traps affected your health, relationships, or well-being?

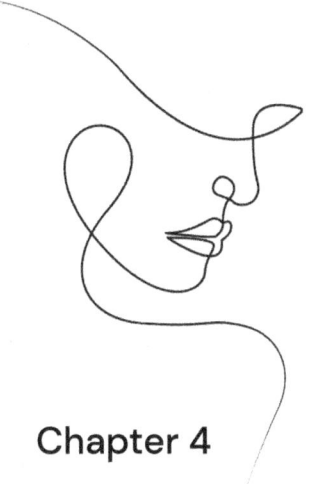

Chapter 4

When the Good Girl Gets Sick

"If you don't know how to say no, your body will say it for you through physical illness."
Dr. Gabor Mate

As a physical therapist, I enjoyed spending my days encouraging my patients and facilitating their potential, but the day I got the call brought me face to face with my habit of serving others at the expense of myself.

"Kate, you have a phone call," the aide whispered to me in the hallway. "Do you want me to take over for you so you can answer it?"

"That's okay. Just ask them to hold, and I'll be right there," I replied as I tightened my grip on the gait belt secured around my patient's waist and returned my attention to encourage her. A few minutes later, I reminded her to reach back for her wheelchair as she unlocked her prosthetic knee and lowered herself down for a well-deserved break. After grabbing her a cup of water, I let the aide know she was ready to go back to her room, made my way into the office, picked up the phone, and listened in a trance as I was given the news of my biopsy results.

I thanked the nurse, hung up the phone, and doubled timed down the hall, flung open the door to the stairwell, skipping steps to get to my next patients' floor, feeling bad that I was late getting to them. As I ran, the conversation swirled in my head, but I pushed it down in the same way I'd suppressed my emotional needs for years, compulsively shifting my attention to the needs of others without taking any time to process my own.

Four hours later, from the privacy of my car, the conversation I'd compartmentalized came flooding back: *Mrs Bartley, your biopsy was positive for papillary thyroid cancer.* That last word floated in my brain like an unwanted guest as I tried to make sense of it being used in the same sentence with my name. It didn't belong, and I wanted to spit it out like spoiled milk you innocently take a swig of before realizing it's bad. I drove down the highway toward my house, trying to figure out a way to keep from bringing it home with me. I wanted to bring home Lawler's Barbeque, not, *Hey, sorry to have to tell you this, but apparently I have cancer.*

As my mind turned it over and over, trying to process the information, my soul started shouting, *No. Please no. I don't want to die. I can't. My kids need me.* I allowed the tears to fill my eyes, obscuring my vision like a windshield fogging up in a rainstorm. As quickly as they came, I swiped them away so I could make it home in one piece, giving me a bit of a reality check. The C word sounded really threatening, but car accidents happen to people every day. Better to stay present and focus on the road than to worry about something intangible.

Later that night, I stood with my back to the fireplace, bracing against it for strength, as I whispered to my husband, "I need to tell you something." I pushed the words out with the same force I'd used to get my son to loosen his grip on the car door on his first day of swim team practice. Those words held fast, just like he did that day, not wanting to face the uncertainty.

When I finally let them out, my husband moved in, wrapping his arms around me, and whispered back, "We'll get through this. It's going to be okay." As he held me, I exhaled my fears with the tension in my body and relaxed into the safety of his embrace.

The following weeks were filled with doctor appointments, scans, surgery, and recovery, and by some miracle, I found time for it all, and the world kept spinning without me.

Why is it always the "Good Girl" who gets cancer?

In one of my favorite Netflix series, *FireFly Lane*, a show about two friends that grow up together, my favorite character, Kate, is diagnosed with breast cancer. I had to stop and replay a scene[6] to catch the connection being depicted between "being good" and getting sick that I'd seen in so many of the shows I'd watched. Deep down, I knew there was some truth to this, but it wasn't something you ever said out loud.

Since my own cancer journey, I'd read several books written by doctors filled with case studies showing this strong correlation and sharing what they kept seeing in their clinics. It always seemed to be the "Good Girl" who got cancer and autoimmune diseases. The main actress, Kate, is depicted as the classic good girl and her costar, Tully, a product of a Hippie mother, plays the "bad" seed of the two. In this same episode, these were the lines that caught my attention: "I don't know how you handle it; being the center of attention all the time; everyone trying to cater to you. It's exhausting. People walking on eggshells around me, worrying about me, and then I can't tell them that I'm scared because then I wouldn't be brave and inspiring."

---

6   *Firefly Lane*, Season 2, Episode 11, Netflix, 2023.

Her friend takes her words in and replies, "I just love you so much," to which Kate responds, "Yeah, that's the hard part."

For many "Good Girls," being on the receiving end of care feels really vulnerable. We aren't used to being in that position, and as much as we want to be loved in that way, our bodies often shrink back from it as if we're being forced to take a spoonful of cod liver oil or something. It's hard to swallow it without feeling like we're taking someone's last ration of food.

Disconnected From Our Feelings

I sit across from caring, empathetic women and hear this same response over and over again: "I have no idea what I want. I can't even define it. I feel so disconnected from my needs and desires. I don't even know how to articulate them. I've always just done what others wanted and needed me to do." I usually have to help them come in the back door by asking what they want less of to get under the rug and find an entryway. They usually say things like...

- I'm tired of being tired all the time.
- I'm tired of feeling so torn.
- I'm tired of being pulled in a million directions and never having time for myself.
- I'm tired of taking on the responsibility for everyone else's well-being.
- It's too much.
- It's heavy.
- I can't do it anymore.
- I'm tired of being lonely.
- I'm tired of crying myself to sleep but muffling the sounds so no one can hear.
- I'm tired of hurting and not knowing what's wrong with me.

- I'm tired of feeling so weak and needy.
- I'm tired of being the person I vowed to never be, hearing myself complain, and being so self-focused.
- I just want to get back to feeling like myself so I can get back to helping others.
- I'm tired of being needed, but at the same time I'm afraid of not being needed anymore.

That clarity makes for a pretty good segue into, "*What would you like instead? What might you be doing differently if you weren't feeling responsible for the whole world?*"

Later in the episode, Kate finally gets in touch with her emotions during a moon ritual as she explores alternative healing methods. Instead of following the guide's suggestion to channel loving energy and express positive affirmations, she trusts her intuition and does what feels right for her. "This is my ceremony, and I'm going to do it my way," she declares, allowing herself to shout out her anger and grief. For the first time, she gets radically honest and lets herself express emotions that had always felt unacceptable. It often takes getting sick to break free from the expectations of how we're supposed to feel and get in touch with what's really happening inside us.

When we grow up hearing messages like...

- "Don't raise your voice at me, young lady."
- "How dare you talk back to me."
- "A woman should be slow to speak, silent in the church, and have words like honey."
- "*Love is patient, love is kind. Put on love above all things.*"

...expressing how you really feel is daunting.

Positive thinking is often the last thing we need to heal. What we need is to get all those pent-up emotions out of us instead of keeping them inside where they're blocking the flow of our energy. We're often trying so hard to be a light for others that we block the waves of that healing love for ourselves. We stay positive and strong, put our own needs on hold, rush down hallways, and skip stairs to guide others into that love until our bodies finally stop us in our tracks and guide us into a position where we can receive it for ourselves. Even then, like Kate, we often deflect it. In one breath, we pray for healing, but in the next, we may unknowingly be sabotaging it.

My goal in this book is not to make a direct correlation between "being good" and chronic illness but to help you see into women's lives and draw your own conclusions, just as many doctors now have. We may not have the capability of drawing labs to prove this, nor do we need to, but we can use our first-hand experiences to see potential roadblocks and open up intuitive pathways to healing. Cancer and disease don't happen in a vacuum but within the contexts of our lives.

When It Doesn't Feel Safe to Step Back

In her book *Risking Rest*, author and OBGYN Carolyn Watts shares the challenges I hear from so many women when it comes to trying to step back from serving others no matter how tired we get:

> "In the past six months, I'd often been the only doctor for 150,000... [until] my body claimed the small luxury of illness.... I'd been working from bed, too sick to stand or sit for long but too driven to rest, anxious to continue doing something, anything, to help."[7]

---

[7] Watts, Carolyn. *Risking Rest: Embracing God's Love Through Life's Uncertainties.* Hope Books, 2023.

Carolyn had been serving in Afghanistan for four years before, like me, her body set a boundary for her and gave her a permission slip. She writes:

> "[I felt] ashamed of having to ask for prayer for the same challenges.... I still find it hard to let people see the mess.... I'd had always managed to keep my mess well hidden.... The exposure of fear felt like failure and the need for help, an admission of terminal defeat, so I kept my heart hidden.... Life, for me, was built on hard work; I knew no other way to live than constant pushing.... My limbs were leaden... my exhausted legs couldn't carry me.... Limits? They were felt but undefined, an edge I was constantly pushing up against but never quite able to locate. I always managed, somehow, to take one step more. Until I couldn't."

Carolyn's story felt so much like my own; only mine was right here in the good ole USA, in a church where everyone was safe. But somehow, the risk of stepping back and the shame of asking for help felt the same.

Carolyn graciously allowed me to interview her about her experience to help me grow in my understanding and ability to support other women struggling in the way she was. I asked, "What did you need when you were dragging yourself up the hills of Afghanistan with nothing left to give?"

She paused, then stated, "I needed someone in authority, someone that was supposed to be protecting me, to say, *'It's okay to step back. Take time for yourself and rest. You matter, too.'* My colleagues and friends were telling me to let them know when I couldn't do it anymore or if I needed anything, but what I really needed was for them to ask, 'What can we do?' I couldn't say it. I couldn't ask. It felt wrong. My calling felt so strong. I thought I had to sacrifice myself."

When you've been taught to follow Jesus, even unto death, speaking up for yourself feels too risky. It doesn't matter if your body is screaming that you're way beyond your human limits and is shutting down in what we call trauma physiology. This is why It's not enough to tell women to reduce their stress and take better care of themselves. It's not that easy. Like Carolyn, we need someone to say, "It's okay to step back. Take time for yourself and rest. You matter, too." Without that reassurance, it takes illness and disease to give us consent, just like it did for me.

Guilt-Free Permission Slip

I'll never forget the freedom I felt when I had doctor's orders to quarantine for a week when I was "radioactive." Part of my treatment to ensure they got any lingering cancer cells that might have been swimming around in my body was to swallow a radioactive iodine pill, and I wasn't supposed to hold my kids near me until the "toxicity" was out of my system. Talk about giving me the security to erect strong boundaries! You need to stay back. I could harm you! That will do it for a woman whose goal in life is to "help" people.

I sat in the middle of my bed that first day, and a wave of confidence washed over me. For the first time in my life, I wasn't questioning what I was supposed to be doing for God. I didn't have to worry if I was in the center of His will or not. I wasn't allowed to be anywhere else but right where I was. It felt like I had this great, big permission slip from God validating my rest, and it said, "Just be right here with me. This is the place I long for you to be." Peace flooded in as I opened up my hands and let go of all the doubts. I found the security I needed to start healing not only my body but the wounds I'd been carrying since childhood. God used that time to rebuild my foundation of trust and teach me what it felt like to receive love without having to do anything for Him or anyone else.

Like a child whose confidence is built on a foundation of secure attachment, a sense of curiosity and excitement arose as I began to explore my desires. I can still feel the smile lifting my cheeks and the expansion of my chest as they formed into words. *I want to use this time to start a blog!* Later that day, I told my husband, and he went out and bought me a laptop. I felt like a kid in a candy shop as I researched, created, and named it "Springing Up." It was a season where God watered me and brought my dry bones back to life. My oldest daughter made me a journal for my birthday that year and stenciled my theme verse on the cover: "The Lord will guide you always; he will satisfy your needs in a sun-scorched land and will strengthen your frame. You will be like a well-watered garden, like a spring whose waters never fail" (Isaiah 58:11). I still have it propped against the light on my desk as an anchor for my soul; a reminder that my needs do matter and how much He longs to satisfy them.

Clearing the Blockages to Healing

When we've spent a lifetime holding back our emotions, dismissing our needs, and trying to be strong for everyone else, it's no wonder our bodies start to break down. In those moments, it's easy to feel frustrated—like our prayers for healing and relief are falling on deaf ears, like God isn't answering. But this isn't about weak faith, and it's not that God isn't listening.

Faith—though powerful and necessary—needs space to flow inward. It's not enough to believe in God, our doctors, and treatments if the effects of that faith can't penetrate the blocks within us—reaching deep into our hearts, cells, and tissues. Healing requires us to clear what's been stuck inside: the grief, anger, fear, and the unconscious beliefs that are driving our distress and dis-ease.

GOOD GIRL RX: Break the Cycle of Self-Neglect

It's easy to dismiss our needs, thinking we can carry on indefinitely, but our bodies know the truth and sound the alarm when we've pushed too far. Instead of seeing these wake-up calls as setbacks, let's view them as opportunities to deepen our awareness and redefine what it means to be strong women. Use these questions as a starting point for reconnecting with your needs and honoring yourself in a way that empowers you to thrive.

Reflection Questions:

1. Where have you noticed similar patterns of disregarding your own needs in favor of serving others? How has this impacted your health or sense of well-being?
2. Have you experienced a "wake-up call" where pain, illness, or exhaustion forced you to stop? What can you learn from that experience? What was the message your body was expressing?
3. If you didn't need to validate your needs, what would you give yourself permission to do today?
4. How can you begin to practice self-compassion and challenge the "Good Girl" conditioning that has led to self-neglect?

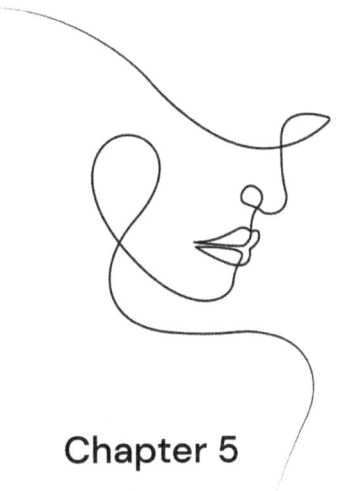

Chapter 5

Learning to Be Good: The Hidden Cost of Praise and Approval

"What gets rewarded gets repeated."
BF Skinner

I always hated being assigned the class monitor. You know, when the teacher gives you the chalk and the authority to write the names on the board of anyone talking while she's gone?

I never wanted to be accused of being the teacher's pet. Being good, for me, was not about trying to kiss up or appear better than everyone else. The last thing I wanted to do was something that would give my classmates reason to hate me. I just wanted to keep the peace and everyone to get along. My intentions for being "good" were pretty clear-cut. When you're good, you get smiles and warm looks of affection, maybe even some special attention. You feel connected. I learned to do what fostered that and avoid the things that didn't.

What We Appreciate, *Appreciates*; Reinforcing Habits Through Praise

When the words "Good Girl" come out of my mouth, I now pause to think about what behaviors I may be reinforcing. I catch myself saying this a lot to my dog. Every time I play ball with her, take her on a walk, or set her food bowl down in front of her after she sits and say "Good girl," I'm reminded how much power those two little words have to form strong habits. I pause and question if I should even be using them, but man, it's hard not to. It's so ingrained as the appropriate thing to say when someone does something you want them to. When I see her sit obediently with "good manners" or bring the ball back that I wanted her to fetch, those words just slip out of my mouth without conscious thought.

Good girl.
Good girl, honey.
Such a good girl.

Message received. Do that again. Do more of that. It will earn me pats on the head, tummy rubs, treats, my bowl of food. Someone will play more ball with me.

How could praising and petting my dog on the head for heeling at my side be a bad thing, you ask? Isn't that the goal? I want my dog to sit and wait patiently for her food. I want her to stop jumping up and down on me and instead sit calmly along my side before I reward her with tossing the ball. I want her to lay down at my feet and let me rub her belly while I watch a show rather than constantly bringing me a ball and begging to play more when I'm tired. Those two words used alongside the things she loves most work wonders! And it worked for me, too. Using words like "good girl," patting a head, and rewarding with treats are really effective strategies for compliant behavior.

I learned that when I did things people liked, I got praised. I received their love and attention, their admiration, their approval and appreciation. I got the very thing that I need most to feel secure in the world: that warm feeling of connection. That's a powerful reward loop for any habit!

What's so wrong with creating habits around that? Isn't that what everyone wants? Absolutely. The problem is that it can lead to an endless loop of trying to do what we perceive *others* want and need in order to get that reward hit. It becomes a vicious cycle of attuning and responding to others in order to feel safely connected to them.

The Reward Loop

I traded in my golden retrievers' harness for a choke collar one day and brought bite size pieces of cheese along on our walk. You should have seen them. They stayed close to my side, continually looking back over their shoulder to check in with me, waiting for validation (cheese) for their next steps. They're usually pulling on their leashes, driven by their curiosity to sniff out every fragrance around them, and moving with a little more pep in their step, but not that day. They were calm, slow moving, and their attention was tuned in to me to make sure they didn't miss out on getting a treat.

You might say, *That's awesome! I wish I could get my dogs to do that! Then I could just enjoy my walk and not have to be pulled by their every whim.* Yes, but the question is, at what cost? The loss of their energy, curiosity, freedom and self leadership.

This type of behavior training can start out as a really good thing. Without a leash, they might get run over. They don't learn boundaries, like where it is okay to poop and where it's not. They might jump up on a child, too eager to greet them, not understanding that a little restraint goes a long way in befriending someone instead of overwhelming them.

This safety patterning and development of boundaries is something we, as parents, rely on to keep our kids protected from danger and help them find their way in a sometimes ruthless world. Please, hear me: I am not advocating that we abandon safety. I'm not saying that conditioning does not have its place. Without it, we may not survive. Having fences around our yards allows our kids to explore and play in safety, and teaching them not to get in a pool until you are in there with them is vital. Learning to listen, attend to our parents, and trust what they say for our good is important. In the context of a loving relationship, feeling safely protected and secure in the world is the very thing that allows us to explore the world with confidence.

God wants this for us, too. He designed us all with built-in safety systems so we can read a room and discern whether or not we need to protect ourselves. Our ability to tune in and sense danger helps us know when to run, when to fight, when to stay quiet and hide, and when to scream out.

Addicted to Appreciation: The Praise Trap

"Good Girls" grow up to be caring moms, loving wives, dependable employees, compassionate therapists, dedicated teachers, and passionate non-profit leaders. They have a gift for seeing when others are struggling, always responding with consideration and empathy. They love big and love well, and we appreciate them for it. They get little notes on their homework from the teacher, great performance reviews, gifts, and cards from others thanking them for all they do. They even have beautiful obituaries written, things like, "She was so selfless. She sacrificed everything for others. She never complained in her last days. She always had a smile on her face. She was always thinking of others."

At first glance, this seems like a beautiful tribute. I mean, who doesn't want to be thought of so highly—so selflessly? It's what we've been taught is the goal in life: to have a servant's heart, be Christlike, and hear "well done, good and faithful servant" when we stand in front of God one day? But the cost is often really, really high. Let's not forget she died. Self-sacrifice always leads to death. There is no denying this natural law of cause and effect. Maybe it's not a literal death, but the slow unraveling of her identity, the quiet ache of loneliness, the death of her dreams, her voice, and her joy. This isn't noble; it's tragic.

It's easy to see this pattern in women's lives, but it's everywhere—even celebrated in our workplaces, communities, and businesses. One day, I was searching for the menu on the website of a restaurant I ate at recently when their mission statement grabbed my attention:

"We approach everything we do with a humble servant's heart — putting the needs of others above our own."

It was a beautiful mission for a business, but as I read through the descriptions of the employees being highlighted, I had to wonder about the impact of all the praise they were receiving. Things like...

> "She consistently exceeds expectations and goes above and beyond."

> "There's nothing she wouldn't do for her team."
> "She truly cares about everyone around her and not about herself."
> "Twenty-four hours a day, she's there to answer the phone, lend an ear, and listen. If there's an emergency, she's the first to respond. Her #1 priority is to help every single one of her teammates grow, personally and professionally."
> "She always has the warmest heart, is always smiling and friendly."
> "Whether it's family, friends, community, teammates, she's always putting others first."

"She's selfless, always putting her time and attention into the growth of others. She sees their potential."

"She gives up her own scheduled hours so others in need can get the work they need, even taking part-time jobs at other businesses just to help out their overworked friends."

"She is always taking care of others, is always there, the first to help out, always putting herself last."

I appreciate going to businesses with well-mannered employees with great customer service! These are all wonderful qualities and ones I want my own children to emulate. The problem is when we're rewarded so lavishly for these "good behaviors," the reward hit can become addictive, leading to imbalance, hidden stress, and chronic self-neglect. *Always* taking care of others, putting yourself last, serving at the expense of yourself, and giving beyond your capacity is not a sustainable way to live.

GOOD GIRL RX: Get Unleashed from the Approval Trap

When we receive praise or approval, it feels natural to feel good. But over time, that appreciation can create a feedback loop where we start depending on others' reactions to feel valued and secure. In the process, we may adjust our actions, words, and even beliefs to maintain that validation, often losing sight of our true needs and desires. Recognizing this pattern is powerful—it gives us a chance to break free, tune into what genuinely matters, and redefine our worth from within. As you reflect on the questions below, consider how freeing it would be to act in alignment with your own values rather than simply responding to what you think others expect.

Reflection Questions:

1. Think of a time when you felt excited and inspired about something you wanted to pursue—maybe a project, dream, or idea that felt important to you. Who did you share it with? How did their response impact you? Did it deflate your hope or give it wings?
2. Reflect on a recent time when someone's praise, approval, or positive feedback made you feel "good." Perhaps it was a compliment from a friend, recognition at work, or a moment of appreciation after helping someone. What actions or behaviors do you find yourself repeating—or avoiding—to hold onto those feelings of approval and acceptance? Jot down your thoughts below.
3. What might shift in your life if you no longer relied on external validation to feel good?

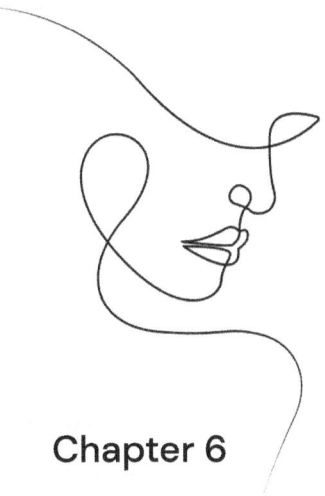

Chapter 6

The Weight of Good Intentions: Going Beyond Our Limits

> *"Empathy without boundaries is self-destructive."*
> Prentis Hemphill

Up until now, I've shared a lot from my own personal journey. But I'm not alone in my struggles. Through the remainder of this book, I'll also be weaving in the stories of other women—those I've interviewed and coached—who have experienced their own versions of the "Good Girl" syndrome. These women's stories reflect the hidden stresses we face as we navigate expectations and how those pressures affect our health, relationships, and self-confidence. One such story is Cathy's, a nurse who poured her heart into caring for others. Cathy found purpose in her work, but behind her selflessness lay a deep sense of emptiness and exhaustion.

Cathy's Story

"I've been a caretaker my entire life, but I don't take good care of myself. I'm tired and peopled out," she confessed.

The weight of responsibility for others' happiness always took precedence over her own well-being. "When I come home, I'm completely spent. It takes me days to recover," she shared. Despite her dedication to caregiving, Cathy harbored unfulfilled aspirations. She had a ministry on the side and dreamed of writing a book, but the fear of rejection held her back. The thought of putting her words out into the world where she could be rejected felt risky and daunting. "I pour, pour, and pour and never receive. I need to learn limits and start saying 'no' to taking on other people's backpacks and people that want things from me," she admitted.

Reflecting on her childhood, Cathy recognized the roots of her caretaking tendencies. Growing up in an alcoholic home, she learned to be hyper-aware of others' moods to ensure her safety. This sensitivity followed her into adulthood, leaving her drained and overwhelmed by the demands of others. "I can tell when someone is upset with me, likes or doesn't like me. I'm super sensitive to it, and I tend to attract people that make it all about them. It's super draining," Cathy shared.

As Cathy embarked on her journey of self-discovery, she grappled with trust and self-acceptance. She longed to step into her true identity and pursue her passions without fear of judgment or failure. "I don't trust myself. I need to learn how to trust myself and walk this out. I can't go out and preach it and teach it if I'm not growing in it personally," she confessed.

But breaking free from old patterns was easier said than done. Cathy found herself saying yes to too many commitments, constantly pushing herself beyond her limits, creating a cycle of chronic fatigue and illness. Cathy lamented, "I say yes to too many things, and it's causing me to miss out on what I really want and feel called to." The fear of rejection and failure loomed large, holding her back from fully embracing the creative pursuits that energized her.

Through her coaching sessions, Cathy learned to set boundaries and prioritize her needs. She discovered the power of self-acceptance and the freedom that comes from letting go of the need to please others. With each breakthrough, Cathy felt a renewed sense of energy and purpose: "I have the ability to shift from feeling anxious to peaceful when I change my thoughts about me, from being unloved to being loved and accepted."

However, old habits die hard, and Cathy faced challenges along the way. Financial struggles and uncertainty threatened to derail her progress, triggering feelings of resentment and fatigue. "I don't know what decision to make. Do we sell the house and move, or should I go back to work to help pay down this debt again?" Cathy agonized. But through it all, she remained committed to her journey, trusting in the process and leaning on her newfound resilience. "I'm working on shifting from, '*What do I do?*' to '*I wonder how God is going to take care of this?*' I need to let go of trying to figure it out and worrying about how my actions will affect everyone else."

Today, Cathy is embracing a new chapter with courage and determination. She completed her book and took bold steps to get it published, overcoming her fear of rejection. She's learning to embrace her "messy me" and share her story vulnerably with the people who need it most, inspiring them to embrace their true selves and live authentically. Cathy's journey serves as a powerful reminder that true healing begins with self-awareness and self-love. By honoring our needs and setting boundaries, we can break free from the cycle of exhaustion and find joy in living authentically.

Boundaries Required: The Cost of Empathy

There is no denying the importance of empathy. It is a God-designed, biological, and psychological response that links us together as humans. It shapes our social behaviors, helps us bond with and nurture our children, and motivates us to make the world a better place. You'd be hard-pressed to find a book or article saying anything negative about it.

We are all made with mirror neurons that allow us to watch someone else, feel what they are feeling, and understand what it's like to be in their shoes. But in order to effectively support them, we have to grasp their reality while maintaining our own sense of self. Empathy can backfire when we lose that balance.

When we get so caught up in another person's emotional experience that we can't distinguish their feelings from our own, we risk being overwhelmed and losing sight of healthy boundaries. Instead of helping, we take on their pain or struggle as if it's our own, and this can sabotage our goal of providing true support.

When empathy turns into over-identification, it activates our protective instincts—causing us to act out of anxiety, fear, or the need to fix. This might lead us to take over someone else's burden, solve their problems for them, or even neglect our own needs in the process. In the end, this sabotages not only our well-being but also the person we're trying to help, as it prevents them from finding their own strength and solutions.

Michael J. Poulin, PhD, an associate professor of psychology at the University of Buffalo, explains the importance of discerning between healthy empathy and hypervigilance: "Overidentifying with someone else's emotions can be stressful, leading to a cardiovascular stress response similar to what you'd experience in the same painful or threatening situation."[8] Feeling another's

---

8   American Psychological Association. "Cultivating Empathy." *Monitor on Psychology*, Nov. 2021, https://www.apa.org/monitor/2021/11/feature-cultivating-empathy.

distress not only wears you out but carrying the emotions of those who are hurting can hurt you.

When we are always feeling everyone else's feelings, it can be hard to have the bandwidth to deal with or even discern our own. Without time and space to get in touch with what is going on within us, they end up simmering underneath, swirling around inside of us like a monster in a cage.

Tammy's Story

Tammy, a middle-aged mother of two adult children on the Autism Spectrum, knew exactly what absorbing the feelings of others was like. We were gently exploring the sensations she was feeling in her body and the emotions connected to them one day, and she could barely allow herself to turn inward to notice them. It didn't feel safe to her. She said, "I can't. There's a monster in there, and if I let it out, it will be *bad*." Meanwhile, she kept having heart arrhythmias, transient ischemic attacks and was on blood pressure medicine. She was scared to death that she was going to die if something didn't change.

As much as she knew she needed to release her emotions to allow her body to regulate, the risk felt too great. It didn't feel safe to unleash all those feelings that had been shoved away for years. Her unconscious mind knew that letting them out could result in shame, criticism, or severe punishment, so it kept a tight lid on them. Keeping them down was how she'd stayed alive. Instead of feeling her own, she learned to read everyone else's emotions so she could respond like a soldier, ready and armed.

One day, after going on a trip to New York, she shared her experience at the World Trade Center site, where the Twin Towers had come crashing down. She said, "Kate, I had to leave and get to a hospital. I became so overwhelmed by pain and grief, and my heart couldn't handle it. I could feel everything those people felt that day, and it was too much. I should have known to prepare myself. I just can't do that anymore."

When we first met, she asked if I was okay working with her because she was not a Christian. She shared how she was an empath and actually wanted to create a website to share tarot card readings and write about things like spiritual healing. I reassured her that she was welcome and this would be a safe, judgment-free space. It was one of my greatest honors to work with her, learn from her, and witness her journey. I have so much more understanding for how the "gift" of empathy is developed and why women with this gift need boundaries around it so they can use their intuitive gifts without having their bodies overwhelmed and shut down from the weight of feeling way more than they were ever intended to.

Nothing Left to Give

Like Cathy and Tammy, I, too, found myself overwhelmed, giving everything to everyone else and struggling to maintain the boundaries needed for my own well-being.

One evening, after walking in from my garage after a long day, a lightbulb of clarity flashed. The exhaustion I was feeling wasn't just physical. It was all-encompassing. I was giving all of myself—my emotional presence, my mental attention, and my physical strength to my patients and their families, and by the time I got home, I had nothing left to give. All I wanted to do was collapse on the couch or go crawl into my bed to numb out and recover. I just needed thirty minutes with a boundary around me, thirty minutes where I wasn't needed, or being pulled in a million directions. Instead, I'd hear my youngest calling, *"Mommy!"* and another voice in my head reminding me that dinner needed to be made.

After dinner, all I wanted was for my husband to take the nighttime duty, but my daughter always wanted me. I'd take a few breaths and muster up the strength, telling myself I could rest alongside her, but when fifteen minutes turned into *one more book, one more time, a little bit longer, one more back rub, please don't go...* and my attempts to be loving were not "enough" for her, I found myself pulling away from the demands and leaving her in tears as I stomped away in a storm of anger, climbed into my bed, and grieved the way it went down. My desire to leave her with butterfly kisses and sweet dreams turned into desperate pleading and her feeling abandoned by me instead.

The part of me that was signaling my need to be off-duty and free from responsibility was disregarded as I pressed on in others regards. It showed up in self-advocacy when it felt the pull for my attention going beyond my energetic capacity. If I had understood my daughter's deep need for attachment security as I do today, and had the awareness to look beyond her clinging behaviors, I might have found the courage to relinquish my sense of duty to everyone else sooner. This would have allowed me the time and energy to replenish myself and be present for her from a place of fullness rather than giving her my leftovers.

I can hear judgment in the voices of other well-meaning Christians trying to preach to me right now, saying, *Well, honey, you were tired because you were depending on your own strength instead of his endless supply. You just need to let go and let God, you know, have more faith. Stop striving. Surrender.* And my advocate is saying, *Why didn't you just let your husband do it? Why didn't you tell someone you felt overextended?* Another part of me is seething and wanting to tell them both to *shut up*. It doesn't feel very understood or appreciated. *Don't they know how weak that would make me look? Don't they know how bad I'd feel if I tried to?*

Symptoms as Messengers

Surrender often comes when we reach the end of ourselves. We can't get there until we feel it. I felt that end through fatigue that stopped me in my tracks, resentment, and anger that cried out to be heard when no one was around. I felt it through abdominal pain that took me to my knees, vertigo that held me captive in my bed. Overwhelm that shut me down and pulled me under the covers. I felt it through TMJ, tension headaches, migraines, and stabbing pain in my feet that not only slowed me down but made it next to impossible to mask the discomfort I was experiencing. It's hard to pretend like you're fine when you grimace with each step. Plantar fasciitis declares to the world on your behalf, *Hey, this lady can't handle another thing!*

My back, my neck, my hips, and the muscles between my shoulder blades took turns echoing the same cry. At least in physical symptoms, we are faced with our limits. It's the things that don't cause pain, like enlarged thyroid nodules, tumors growing in the dark, and rising inflammatory markers that pose the greatest risk. We can keep going with them. They can be ignored... at least until they can't anymore. I'd feel the pain and seek relief through ice, heat, ibuprofen–whatever brought it the fastest. I'd lift my butt off the seat, put inserts under my feet, and use all kinds of avoidance tactics to anything that might aggravate it. Well, except for helping others that is–that was off the table. People needed me. And deep down, if I'm being honest, it made me feel good about myself... or at least, not so bad.

My chosen method was whatever provided the quickest avenue back to doing all the things. It became like a ping pong game: symptom, relief, new symptom, relief, longer lasting symptom, shorter period of relief, illness, a little respite, back to work, and the pattern continued. As it did, I grew increasingly frustrated with my body, feeling betrayed by it. We know cognitively that saying no is the solution for when we've reached our physical limits and are overextending ourselves, but that bypasses our fears and fails to acknowledge the vulnerable parts of our soul that don't feel safe enough to step back, ask for help, or give ourselves permission.

Relief is not the answer. That is a flight response to avoid what we're feeling. The key to healing is learning to embrace vulnerability and sit with the discomfort of needing and receiving rather than trying to escape it. It's not easy and often requires support and resources to navigate the deep insecurity and anxiety that arise when we can no longer rely on our coping mechanisms of self-sufficiency and caretaking. But oh, the life that awaits when we find the courage to move through fear and discomfort and create meaningful change!

Respecting Our Limits

I feel really awful about the number of older women I used to make lie on a mat table with only one pillow under their neck, explaining that it wasn't good for them to have more support and that they needed to rest in "good" alignment. I finally realized at age 45 that was really crappy advice. After years of lying on a really firm mattress that my husband and I bought cheap for the guest room, my pain became greater than my guilt, and I finally agreed to spend money on a new one. For twenty years, I'd been forcing my body to rest at its end ranges instead of supporting it and respecting its limits. That's like forcing your Barbie Doll to do the straddle splits when her body isn't made to do that. When we push ourselves past our end ranges, our bodies eventually start hollering at us.

If you've ever used a ponytail holder one too many times and felt it snap in your hands, you understand the principle of respecting limits. When we ignore our body's signals and push beyond its capabilities, we risk breaking down completely. Just like the rubber band escapes use when the materials finally break down, our bodies provide a way out for us when we exceed our limits. When we respect our limits and honor our boundaries, we maintain our integrity and prevent ourselves from ending up in the trash can, feeling useless. This practice ensures we stay strong and capable, avoiding the pitfalls of overextension.

GOOD GIRL RX: Respect Your Limits

True empathy and care start with honoring our own limits and understanding that we can only support others sustainably out of an overflow of the love we first receive. Take a moment to reflect on the questions below and consider what shifts you might make to create more balance, respect your boundaries, and embrace self-compassion on your journey.

Reflection Questions:

1. Do you have the "gift" of empathy? Do you find yourself being hyper-aware of others' moods and easily drained or overwhelmed by them? What has been the price of empathy for you?
2. When have you felt completely spent, with nothing left to give? How does your body signal to you that it's time to be "off-duty?" What gets in the way of honoring that? What might you need to let go of?
3. If I asked your body to rate how respected and cared for it felt by you, on a scale of 1-10, what would it say?

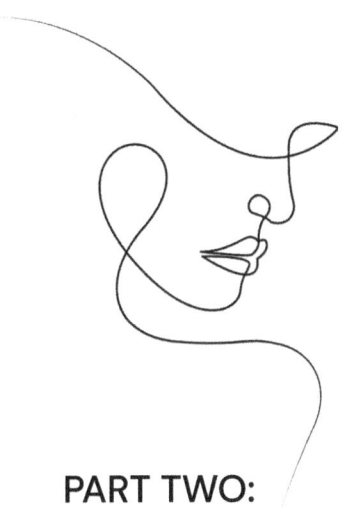

PART TWO:

THE GOOD GIRL WHO BEGAN TO UNDERSTAND HER BODY

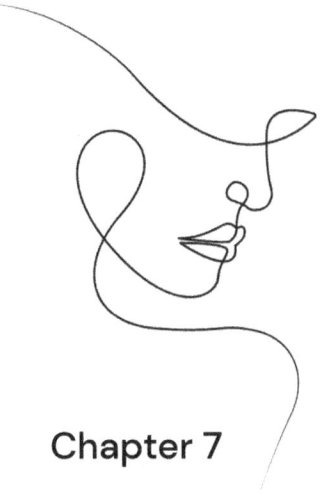

Chapter 7

When Normal Doesn't Feel Normal: Understanding and Healing the Body's Trauma Responses

"Our autonomic nervous system is always working on our behalf, listening to the world around us and within us, and sending messages of safety or warning."
Deb Dana[9]

A Body That Wouldn't Calm Down

I should have been getting better. That's what they told me. "You'll be back to normal in a week." Instead, nothing felt normal. My heart raced just standing in the kitchen making scrambled eggs that morning, and climbing the stairs to my bedroom felt

---

9   Idea as presented in: Dana, Deb, and Stephen W. Porges. *The Polyvagal Theory in Therapy: Engaging the Rhythm of Regulation*. W. W. Norton & Company, 2018.

like scaling a mountain—halfway up, I had to stop to catch my breath. *This isn't normal.* My body wasn't bouncing back, and nothing about the way I felt *felt* safe.

My inner protector was analyzing the storm going on inside of me, going through worst-case scenarios. *What's wrong with my heart? Why can't I catch my breath? Why am I feeling so weak? What if this is a pulmonary embolism?* Google was the opposite of helpful. Instead of providing reassurance, it just amplified everything. Pulmonary embolism? *"Get to the ER immediately. This can be fatal if untreated."* And then, as if the chaos inside wasn't enough, the news announced a tornado watch for later that day. The forecast seemed to echo my internal turbulence, amplifying my spiraling fears. *What if I need to go to the hospital and can't get there? What if the roads are blocked? What if something bad happens and I'm alone?*

I called my doctor's office, desperate for answers, only to hear, "The office is closed. He's already gone for the day." The nurse was kind, listened to what was going on, and managed to squeeze me in for a last-minute EKG at an outpatient imaging center. I drove myself to the clinic, whispered silent prayers, and tried to stay calm as electrodes were stuck to my chest. A few minutes later, I got my answer. "Everything is normal. Your heart looks fine."

Normal? My body begged to differ.

When "Normal" Doesn't Feel Safe

I find it funny that we use the word "normal" to describe something that the body identifies as everything *but* normal, with no explanation for our symptoms. We go home with no answers and are expected to just relax, go to sleep, and get on with our life when the body is stuck in fight or flight. Hearing that my heart was okay and ruling out an embolism brought some relief, but it still didn't explain, validate, or mirror what I was experiencing. Nothing about what I was feeling felt normal.

An hour later, I was hunkered down in the kitchen closet with my kids, holding pillows over our heads while the wind roared and branches cracked outside. I should've felt relief when the tornado missed our neighborhood by a mile, but I still had one swirling inside of me.

Now I know why my body responded the way it did in the movie theatre years later. Those physical sensations—shortness of breath and tightness in my chest—were far too familiar. They were the same ones I felt in the days after surgery, huddled in fear as the tornado passed over us. My nervous system had filed that memory away, labeled it *dangerous,* and vowed to keep me away from anything that resembled it. My body didn't care whether I or someone else labeled them harmless. My nervous system viewed them as dangerous. *We've experienced this before. It wasn't safe. Get out!*

The Body's Silent Warning System

Our bodies are brilliant. Without us even realizing it, our autonomic nervous system (ANS) scans for signs of safety or danger. When it senses a threat—whether real or not—it mobilizes us to respond. That's what happened to me. My heart raced, blood rushed to my core, and my body prepared to get away from the threat. It's a reflex, as automatic as putting your arm out in front of your child when you have to stop the car suddenly.

The problem? My body wasn't responding to the *present moment* but the *past.* And in trying to ignore, resist, and *will* it away-I was suppressing my body's natural way of discharging that activation energy. It wasn't until I finally told my husband what was happening and let him take me to the hospital that the energy began to move through me in the form of the "shakes."

Why Trauma Responses Linger

Trauma isn't about the event itself; it's about how our body experienced it. If we go through something overwhelming—without someone there to sit with us, hold us, or help us process it—our nervous systems hold onto it. Those unprocessed experiences become stored within us. We might not remember them consciously, but our bodies do. They shape how we react to new situations, like the harmless indigestion that sent me into a panic.

This is why two people can experience the same event but have entirely different responses. One might shake it off; the other might carry it for years.

The difference often lies in:

- Whether someone was there to help us feel safe,
- Our past experiences with fear, uncertainty or helplessness, and
- How overwhelmed our nervous system already felt.

When our body stays stuck in survival mode, we don't just feel anxious or overwhelmed. We get sick. Symptoms like panic attacks, insomnia, hormone imbalances, and chronic fatigue start to show up. That's what happened to me after surgery. My body didn't return to "normal" because I was stuck in a trauma response with no understanding of how to process my experience or that I needed to.

From Survival to Safety

Healing begins when we learn to understand what's happening inside us—when we listen to the signals our body is sending and decode the message in them. That day during the storm, my heart raced, my breath felt shallow, and the uncertainty swirled in my chest like an invisible storm of its own, but I didn't tell anyone. I didn't cry out for help or let my husband see how scared I was. I was the strong one—the one who didn't need anything. So I tucked it all away and tried to function, focussing on what needed to be done. That's what strong women do, right? We soldier through. We dismiss the alarms our body is raising and tell ourselves it's "no big deal."

But it was a big deal.

The medication I'd been prescribed after surgery had pushed me into hyperthyroidism—something my body sensed long before it was confirmed. My nervous system was already in overdrive, reacting to the very real threats of an invasive surgical procedure and a cancer diagnosis. It wasn't just my body recovering from surgery—it was also navigating the stress of what I'd been through and that matters. The adrenaline and cortisol surging through my system in the wake of the operation likely heightened my body's sensitivity to the thyroid medication. My nervous system was already in fight-or-flight, and that elevated metabolic state made what might have been a 'normal' dose react abnormally.

This isn't something we talk about enough, but it's critical for medical professionals to take into account the context a woman's body is in after surgery—her nervous system state, her stress levels, and her history. Without understanding those other factors, we can get into a game of chasing symptoms and constantly adjusting medications without addressing the full picture. When the body is already on high alert, even well-intentioned treatment can exacerbate things.

My body was doing its best to protect me, but unresolved stress and overwhelm got stored away. And years later, when those same sensations returned—shortness of breath, chest pressure, and that uneasy feeling—it all came rushing back. My body remembered. That's the thing about trauma—it isn't just about what happened. It's about how our body remembers it and how alone we felt when it was happening.

For years, I didn't let myself feel the full weight of those moments. I didn't cry. I didn't let anyone see my fear, not even myself. But my body bore witness to it. When we keep holding it all in, it doesn't go away—it waits. It waits for a moment to surface, to be felt, to be released. That moment came for me years later, during a business mastermind of all places, when the dam I'd been holding back finally broke.

Healing Trauma

I was sitting in a mastermind training one day and got really emotional during the call. I was working on filling in the blanks on a worksheet to help me better articulate what I do as a coach, and this is what flooded out of me:
You will no longer struggle with...

The fear of dying
The fear of never being healthy again
The fear of always feeling this way
Feeling like no one understands
Feeling like there is no one you can call for help.
Feeling alone in what you are going through.
Feeling like you are stuck in a situation you desperately want out of
Feeling like God is not answering your cries for help

When I got off the call, I curled myself in a ball in my closet, called my sister to process it, and then allowed myself to really cry. As I did, my body started trembling and shaking as it had done after childbirth and my panic attack in the ER. I don't think I'd ever let myself really cry about how scared I'd been all those times, but man, did my body remember it all vividly.

What I'm realizing now is that this was about so much more than being diagnosed with cancer or becoming hyper-vigilant of every symptom as a potential threat of recurrence. It was about trauma.

I used to judge people I thought of as "hypochondriacs," but now I have so much more compassion. Someone doesn't just decide to worry about their health. It's a side effect of one too many life-threatening experiences.

As I sat trying to process all that was flooding back, I started writing about all the times I'd felt alone, unseen, and unheard when I was experiencing something scary.

- The time I couldn't breathe after giving birth to my son, pressing the call button in panic while the nurse stood there asking questions instead of helping me.
- The day of my biopsy, when I went alone and felt the flood of emotion hit afterward as the nurse asked, "Where's your ride?"
- The nights I lay in bed, my fingers pressed to my wrist, silently taking my pulse and thinking, *What if my heart stops and I don't wake up?* careful not to let my husband see.

These experiences weren't just about what happened. It's about how alone I felt while they were happening. When we don't have someone attuning to us, witnessing us, or helping us feel safe, those moments leave their mark on our nervous system. Fear becomes terror. Vulnerability becomes helplessness. Our bodies hold onto that stress, storing it away like unfinished business.

Trauma responses are not a choice but the body's instinctual reaction to danger—whether real or perceived. Just as your leg shoots out when a doctor taps your knee with a reflex hammer, your nervous system responds to cues of danger before you even think about it. The longer the nervous system stays stuck in a state of heightened alert without returning to a sense of safety, the more those stress responses take a toll. Anxiety, insomnia, panic attacks, hormone imbalance, crashing fatigue, and inflammation are just a few of the ways it can show up in the body. Our body isn't broken; it's communicating. It's asking for the care, safety, and space it needs to release what it's been holding.

Looking back, my body wasn't just reacting to hyperthyroidism or post-op recovery—it was carrying years of unresolved fear, stress, and the emotional imprints of loneliness and disconnection. And when my nervous system couldn't hold it anymore, it sounded the alarm again and again. This is the true trauma: not just the frightening experience itself, but the silence we hold around it. The shame. The self-reliance. The belief that we should be strong enough to handle it-alone.

But here's the good news: survival strategies that once protected us can be unlearned. Healing begins when we finally listen and respond with compassion to what our body is trying to tell us.

The Four Survival Strategies

Trauma—whether brief or prolonged—impacts each of us differently. How we respond depends on many factors: our childhood experiences, attachment patterns, and the ways we learned to navigate conflict, fear, or pain. From a young age, we develop instinctual survival strategies to cope, favoring the responses that best kept us safe or helped us avoid further harm. These patterns, while protective at the time, can follow us into adulthood, complicating our ability to heal, build healthy relationships, and feel confident and secure in the world.

Understanding these instinctual responses has been incredibly freeing for me. Gaining clarity around my own patterns gave me the self-compassion I needed to start changing them. My hope is that this section will do the same for you. The more awareness we bring to these automatic responses, the more confidence we gain to interrupt them, reclaim choice, and move toward the healing and freedom we long for.

There are four primary responses our nervous system uses to protect us in the face of danger: *fight, flight, freeze, and fawn.*

- **Fight** is our instinct to stand our ground and confront a threat.
- **Flight** drives us to escape or run away to find safety.
- **Freeze** immobilizes us, like an animal playing dead, or gives us time to pause, disconnect, and figure out our next move.
- **Fawn**—the less commonly known response—causes us to appease or please the threat as a way to diffuse harm and secure safety.

You've likely experienced some or all of these responses at different times in your life. They're automatic, designed to protect us. But when we stay stuck in these survival strategies—repeating the same patterns we leaned on in childhood—they can hold us back from truly living, loving, and thriving.

In the following chapters, I'll share personal stories and examples to illustrate how each response—*fight, flight, freeze, and fawn*—shows up in our lives. Together, we'll explore what keeps us stuck in survival mode, what these patterns are trying to protect, and how we can begin to shift toward a healthier, more embodied way of being.

GOOD GIRL RX: Decode Your Body's Messages

When we shift from seeing symptoms as something to eliminate to viewing them as invitations to uncover our body's wisdom, we gain the opportunity to understand our true needs and heal from past experiences. A dose of curiosity and compassion can be the most powerful medicine, strengthening trust and building a supportive relationship with your body—one that honors both its natural healing capacity and your ability to interpret its messages without adding fear. The best part? This medicine comes without unwanted side effects!

Reflection Questions:

1. Have you ever been told that everything was 'normal' when it didn't feel normal to you? How did that experience make you feel? What did you need to hear instead?
2. When you notice a symptom or discomfort, do you respond with curiosity, frustration, or fear? What might shift if you started seeing these sensations as friendly signals rather than threats or annoyances?
3. What objections arise when you consider listening to your body's signals instead of pushing through, overriding, or resisting them? What is one way you could start relating to your body in a way that cultivates more assurance and support?

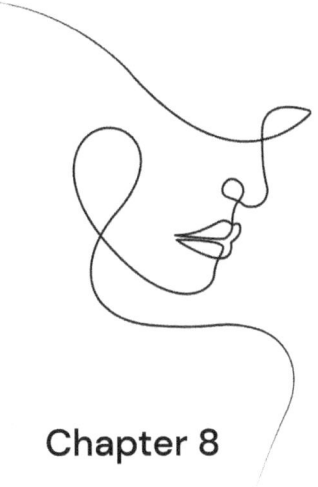

Chapter 8

Running for Peace: Escaping Discomfort Through the Flight Response

---

"Anxiety is contagious... When we flee from it, we not only abandon ourselves, we perpetuate the disconnect."
Harriet Lerner[10]

"I've been so stressed about my marriage that it's starting to affect my body. My stomach's been in knots, just like when I was a kid, and I'm dealing with anxiety again for the first time in years. My whole body feels tense like it's bracing for something bad to happen, and I honestly don't know what's next between us."

---

10 Ideas as presented in: Lerner, Harriet. *The Dance of Fear: Rising Above Anxiety, Fear, and Shame to Be Your Best and Bravest Self.* HarperCollins Harper Perennial, 1990.

A client of mine was painting a vivid picture of how our bodies mirror our conflicts, reflecting the emotional and relational distress we so often experience. I got curious and asked, "What did you need to know as a little girl when you felt this way? What does the part of you that's feeling anxious need right now?"

She paused, then replied, "It's scared. It feels so uncertain."

To help her connect with what was happening in her body, I asked, "What does your body want to do right now?"

"It wants to run," she said. "To leave and get away. I just want to feel peace, freedom, and safety—or shut down because I'm so tired of fighting."

I sent her an audio exercise designed to work with the flight response and restore her sense of safety. About thirty minutes later, she texted back: "Well, that helped a lot. I can breathe easier. Thank you."

During her next session, we talked about the experience. "I'd been running around anxious when you sent it," she explained. "So, I pulled into a Walmart parking lot and did it twice. Everything shifted afterward, and this calmness came over me. I really needed that."

She continued, "I've always thought of myself as a runner, like I was weak or couldn't deal with conflict. But now I have so much more understanding and compassion for myself. As a kid, I couldn't escape the conflicts in my home. I couldn't run away—our nearest neighbors lived a mile away, and there was nowhere safe to go. So, I'd fight and scream, or I'd sit in the driveway, hide in the truck, or go numb on the couch in the formal living room. I'd sit so still they'd walk right past me, not even realizing I was there.

"When I got married, it was the same. I couldn't run away from conflict with my husband because we had a baby, so I fought and shouted just like I had as a kid. Running wasn't an option. I felt trapped." She smiled as she recalled the exercise. "During it, I climbed up on this imaginary rock, and for the first time, I felt safe. I could breathe. I could see clearly. The stress left my body, and I thought, *Okay, I can think now.* When my husband came home later, I was fine—not because I'd given up, but because I was calm."

Running Away From Home

My client's experience takes me back to the day I was at a breaking point with my mother and announced I was leaving. I packed a bag and started walking down the street in my neighborhood, feeling empowered. I got all the way to McDonald's, and sat licking my 25-cent ice cream cone before reality set in, and that power I felt moments before deflated. I had to go back. A grown-up might call my homecoming "repentance," like the prodigal child return, but my pivot that day didn't feel like a win, but a resignation. It felt like being forced to shake your opponent's hand when you've been defeated. A true win would have been being met with arms of love when I got home–a listening ear and desire to hear what made me feel so threatened that I needed to escape.

That's exactly what my client experienced that day as she took herself through this exercise. It wasn't giving up. She learned how to give her younger self the reassurance and safety she needed in the midst of conflict and uncertainty. She met herself the way she'd needed in the past. Healing is always a byproduct of repair.

Stress and conflict are part of being human, living in the world with other humans, and very real threats. We're not always going to handle conflict well as children or parents, but oh, how wise our bodies are to help us navigate through it.

I'm glad no one stopped me when I left home. I needed to let that energy move through my body. I needed to know I could get away from conflict if I needed to. When we can't, that flight energy gets trapped in the body as anxiety. When I think back to the times in my life when I started struggling with anxiety and panic attacks for the first time, that's exactly what was going on. I felt stuck in my life, trapped by what I perceived as "inescapable" circumstances.

We don't have to be victims of sex trafficking or in an abusive marriage where our lives are in jeopardy for our bodies to respond like we are. All it takes is the perception that we can't "get away" or create change for our survival instincts to be activated.

My client realized what she was feeling in her stomach that day was the same feeling she had as a child when she was scared in the midst of conflict in her home. Her body just did what it needed to do to keep her safe. It was safer for her to fight back when she was being threatened verbally, and when that didn't work and getting away wasn't an option, she shut all that "escape" energy down and collapsed on the couch or in her truck. That activation energy we feel in our bodies is often an old alarm rooted in our early childhood experiences.

Dr. Russell Kennedy, author of *Anxiety Rx*, describes anxiety as not just a mental state but a survival-based alarm that originates in the body.[11] The feelings of tightness, nausea, or unease we experience are often echoes of unresolved emotional pain stored in the nervous system. My client wasn't just anxious about the present moment—her body was replaying a familiar threat that had been imprinted in childhood. There are many books and teachings designed to help us 'think' our way out of anxiety and get back to the peace that passes all understanding, yet so many women remain trapped in its grip. That's because anxiety isn't something we can break free from through mental efforts alone. To truly heal, we must address the alarm where it lives: in the body.

---

11   Kennedy, Russell. *Anxiety Rx: A New Prescription for Anxiety Relief from the Doctor Who Created It*. Lioncrest Publishing, 2020.

I tested this with a friend recently and had her replay the last time she felt anxious. She stated, "My stomach drops, then my mind starts spiraling, and my chest gets tight."

Her body sensed something in her world and responded to it at a visceral level, *then* her mind went to work to try and figure out what to do to restore her peace. Her mind began searching, analyzing, and ruminating, trying desperately to figure out what she'd done wrong and how she could remedy it. How did her body know to feel that dread? It read cues of danger in her environment and rang the fire alarm, just like it did when she was a little girl, implementing the same self-preservation habits that worked to keep her safe the first time. The problem was that those strategies were outdated. Instead of bringing her peace, they were amplifying her anxiety and making it really hard to be present and authentic with the people she loved most.

This same pattern played out in my own life at a women's conference, where the alarm bells of my nervous system took me back to old, familiar stories of rejection and disconnection.

Triggered at a Women's Conference

A few years ago, I attended a women's conference centered on the theme of togetherness—something I longed for more of but often struggled to experience in the walls of the church. I came in hopeful, ready to move past the patterns that had blocked me in the past, reminding myself *I've come a long way. I'm not going to get upset when they talk about this today. I can lean in instead of getting activated and running away.*

I enjoyed the conference speakers and was excited about embracing change, so I stepped forward for prayer at the end, desiring accountability and a breakthrough. I also wanted guidance on how to use my gifts without falling back into old patterns of leading in isolation. I needed a space where I could connect and contribute and experience healthy interdependency.

I intentionally chose an older woman from another church, hoping she might understand my struggles better, but the room was loud, and I had to keep repeating myself, which made it hard for her to hear my heart. She did her best and prayed for me, asking that I rest, heal, and receive love—beautiful sentiments, but they didn't address the deeper longing I was trying to express. I didn't want more rest; I wanted to do what the speaker's message encouraged: contribute my gifts as a part of the body, working together, side by side. I was ready!

Instead of feeling encouraged and filled with hope, I walked away feeling misunderstood and frustrated, and as I left the auditorium, my body went into panic mode. The old stories started replaying: *No one understands. No one gets it. Things are never going to change. You'll never be able to use your gifts alongside others and experience that togetherness. They don't even want you. Who are you to think you have anything to offer, anyway?*

I knew what was happening, and I didn't want to leave with that familiar storm raging within me. I was determined to do things differently this time. I forced myself to slow down and stood in the lobby, scanning for someone else to talk to, someone who might be able to listen and provide a corrective experience. Instead, my brain found reinforcements for the narrative: *There's no one to help you here. No one cares. They are all busy talking to each other. Just go.*

I fled to my car, climbed inside, and let the tears fall. This time, though, instead of spiraling into the old stories, I paused, placed my hand on my chest, slowed my breathing, and sent compassion to my younger self. Once the activation dialed down, I scanned my mind for someone I could reach out to before driving away and remembered a woman I'd met recently at a small group coaches meeting. She was new to the church, and after realizing we had some things in common, I'd invited her to lunch, where she opened up about her own experiences with church hurt. Believing she was a safe person who could understand what I was going through, I took a deep breath and called her. She listened compassionately, and we agreed to meet for lunch the following week, providing the glimmer of hope my body needed to settle into peace.

How I Calmed My Flight Response

Making that call was a turning point. Sharing my experience with someone who understood helped replace the danger signals in my nervous system with cues of safety. My body was able to release the arousal energy, and my flight response calmed. I drove home not just with relief but with a thread of connection.

When I met with her the next week, we uncovered a wound I thought I had healed but was still being triggered. It went back to my time at the church plant, where my closest friend had stepped into a busy and demanding season of life. Her husband became the pastor, and she returned to full-time work to support their family. She poured herself into building relationships at work and inviting people to church, which was beautiful to see. But every time we crossed paths, she was deeply engaged in conversations with others. She'd give me a quick pat on the shoulder or a kind compliment like, "What you're doing is so important," and though her words were well-meaning, I didn't feel valued- I felt invisible.

Over time, her words and actions reinforced a painful belief I had carried since childhood: *People are too busy with others' needs to have time for you. You matter less.* This wasn't about just her actions—it was an echo of early imprints that had stayed with me, and the church plant experience reinforced it: *Others' needs are more important.*

Looking back, I can see how this dynamic played out in countless ways. On Sundays, I'd look around, longing to connect, but the people I wanted to talk to were always focused on ministering to someone else. I'd wait, hoping they'd eventually look up and become available, but it rarely happened. Instead, if I wanted to connect, I had to initiate it, tapping them on the shoulder and offering a quick hug as they moved on to their next conversation. Every time it happened, it only served to confirm my deep sense of rejection.

Over time, this pattern became a trigger for my flight response. It felt safer to pull away and retreat into self-reliance than to sit with the sting of rejection. To avoid the pain, I began seeking out others who seemed open and ready for connection—scanning the room for someone else that was sitting alone. While this shift allowed me to move toward healthier dynamics, I struggled to fully experience mutuality even then. I often found myself slipping back into familiar patterns, focusing on helping others connect while neglecting my own emotional needs. Instead of showing up fully for myself, I was unconsciously abandoning the little girl within me, reinforcing her rejection story like a broken record. Her longing for more authentic, interdependent relationships with other women remained unmet as I mirrored the habits of connection I had learned growing up.

Recognizing Trauma Reenactments

As I reflected, I realized this wasn't just a coincidence—it was a pattern I'd been drawn to repeatedly, like a trauma reenactment. I was unconsciously placing myself in environments where the same dynamics played out, as though seeking a corrective experience, but instead, the same imprints replayed: *Others' needs come first. Your emotional needs aren't a priority. If you want to connect, be helpful.*

This realization helped me see that my flight response wasn't about weakness or failure—it was a survival strategy my body had learned long ago. But now, I could begin to choose differently. By recognizing the narrative at play and taking small steps—like reaching out in vulnerability to my new friend instead of pulling away and isolating—I started to rewrite the story.

When Flight Feels Safer Than Staying

The flight response isn't always as obvious as running from rejection or conflict. Often, it takes on subtle forms of avoidance, allowing us to escape discomfort without even realizing it. This response doesn't just show up in relationships or external stressors—it also plays out in how we relate to our own bodies and physical sensations. Here are some common ways it can manifest:

- **Overworking:** Throwing yourself into work to avoid emotions or conflicts.
- **Busyness:** Filling your day with nonstop tasks or errands to stay distracted.
- **Helping Behaviors:** Redirecting your focus to others, using care for them as a way to avoid sitting with your own feelings of rejection or inadequacy.
- **Choosing Self-Reliance Over Reaching Out:** Opting for independence instead of asking for help to protect yourself from the vulnerability of unmet needs.
- **Pulling away to avoid rejection:** isolating yourself from connection to shield against the risk of rejection.
- **Ghosting:** Avoiding conversations or situations by cutting off communication rather than addressing the discomfort directly.
- **Hyper-focusing on Productivity:** Pouring yourself into accomplishments to feel in control or to suppress feelings of inadequacy.
- **Escaping Through Exercise:** Using physical activity excessively as a way to release tension and avoid sitting with emotions.

- **Binge or Emotional Eating:** Turning to food or alcohol as a form of self-soothing, comfort, or reward, often using it as a way to numb your emotions and avoid the deeper unmet needs.
- **Health Fixation:** Seeking safety through relentless doctor visits, researching, or rigidly adhering to health protocols in an effort to escape feelings of vulnerability and uncertainty. These actions may provide a sense of control but often reinforce messages of threat and fragility.
- **Managing Discomfort Through Avoidance**: Engaging in strategies like excessive stretching, over-relying on ice or heat, or avoiding activities altogether in an attempt to escape sensations of pain or discomfort. While these actions can be supportive, they often stem from a state of activation rather than agency, reinforcing the idea that your body's sensations are unsafe and something to 'get away from.'
- **Compulsive Cleaning or Organizing:** Creating order in your environment to feel in control when emotions feel chaotic.
- **Over-planning or Constant Scheduling:** Avoiding uncertainty by rigidly planning every detail of your day or life.
- **Geographical Escaping:** Feeling the urge to move houses, travel, or "start fresh" to leave behind discomfort.
- **Perfectionism:** Constantly refining, fixing, or improving things to avoid criticism, gain approval, or suppress feelings of inadequacy.
- **Pacing or Restlessness:** Physically moving, pacing, or fidgeting as an outlet for built-up anxiety.
- **Overthinking and Ruminating:** Replaying conversations, obsessing over "what-ifs," and running through every possible scenario to avoid the uncertainty or

emotional risk of making a decision or facing an unknown outcome.
- **Outsourcing Decisions:** Delegating choices to others to avoid the emotional risk or accountability of making the "wrong" decision.

These subtle forms of flight may provide temporary relief, but they often come at a cost. They allow us to escape the immediate discomfort, yet they also perpetuate the very patterns we long to get away from. They keep us running from the very things that need our care and attention. By tuning into your body's signals and responding with care, you can create a way of escape that doesn't reinforce messages of threat but instead leads to peace and healing.

When Flight Is Appropriate vs Sabotaging

Not all flight responses are harmful. Sometimes stepping away is the wisest choice—whether to avoid escalating conflict, calm your nervous system, or regain clarity. The key difference is agency vs activation. When we consciously choose to walk away, it supports our well-being and creates space for reflection. But when flight is reactive- driven by old wounds and conditioned fears rather than present needs- it often sabotages our ability to stay present, work through discomfort, and feel truly seen.

What Are We Trying to Escape?

When the flight response is triggered, we're often trying to get away from:

- Pressure, demands, or expectations that feel too heavy to carry.
- Hard conversations we'd rather avoid.

- The pain of being misunderstood, unseen, or rejected.
- Accountability for decisions or actions we're not ready to face.
- Vulnerability—the discomfort of being present with sensations or emotions that feel overwhelming or threatening, whether physical or emotional.

The problem is, while running can feel safer at the moment and might even bring a fleeting sense of relief, it doesn't provide the lasting or true peace we're longing for. Avoidance creates a false sense of safety by temporarily removing us from conflict or threat, but it doesn't resolve the underlying issue. Instead, it often amplifies the very things we're trying to escape—leaving us stuck in a cycle of fear, avoidance, and disconnection.

True peace isn't found in running away from discomfort; it's found in moving toward resolution with courage and self-compassion. Momentary relief through avoidance keeps us hiding—from the life, relationships, and growth we deeply desire. Lasting peace comes from learning to face what feels unsafe with the confidence that we can handle it, process it, and come out stronger on the other side.

Learning to Stay With Yourself

I've had to learn how to pause, notice, and gently question my flight instincts instead of following them on autopilot. Here are some things that have helped me:

Pause and Breathe: When you feel the urge to flee, take a moment to slow down. Put a hand on your heart and shift your attention to your breath, using it to ground yourself, noticing the air moving in and out and the rise and fall of your ribcage.

Get Curious: Notice the sensations in your body and ask yourself: *Does this feel familiar? Is this a present threat or an echo of the past? What am I trying to escape?* These simple questions can help you pause and bring awareness to what's happening. Curiosity softens the fear response in your brain and allows your rational mind to re-engage, helping you distinguish between what's real and what might be an old story replaying.

Offer Compassion: Imagine speaking to yourself as you would a friend: *It makes sense that you want to run. This is hard. But you're not alone—you can stay with yourself here.*

Stay Present: Sometimes, staying doesn't mean fixing the problem. It means simply staying with yourself through the discomfort, letting it move through your body without taking action to get away from it.

Why It Matters

When we begin to work through these patterns, we reclaim the connection we've been longing for—not just with others but with ourselves. Each time you pause, breathe, and stay with the discomfort, you're rewriting the story. You're showing yourself that you don't have to run anymore. You shift from self-abandonment to becoming your biggest supporter and advocate. And by staying, you create space for the peace, connection, and belonging you've been seeking all along.

GOOD GIRL RX: Stay With Yourself

When your flight response is activated, it's your body signaling that something feels unsafe. Instead of running or abandoning yourself, choose to stay present and connected. Healing begins here—by grounding in your body, breathing through the discomfort, and allowing the activation to move through you. This doesn't mean you have to stay in the space or situation where you feel unsafe. Staying with yourself is about choosing agency—stepping away if needed, creating the safety your body is asking for, and responding with intention instead of reacting from a place of anxiety.

Reflection Questions:

1. Think about a recent conflict or stressful situation where you felt the urge to escape or withdraw. What physical sensations or emotions did you notice in your body at that moment? How did you respond to the feeling of wanting to "run away?"
2. Take a moment to look back at the list of ways the flight response can show up in our lives—overworking, isolating, redirecting to helping behaviors, overthinking, binge eating, and others. Which of these resonate most with you? Write them down or name them quietly to yourself.
3. What might these strategies be trying to protect you from?
4. What is one small step you could take to pivot from these patterns the next time you notice them? How could you pause, ground yourself, and meet your needs with compassion rather than self-sabotage?

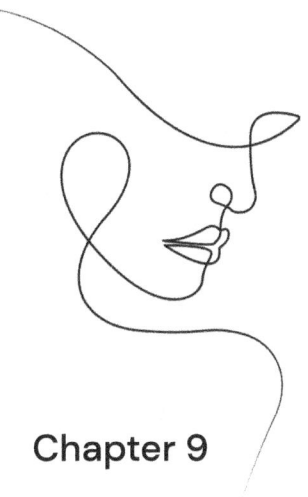

Chapter 9

Unleashing Her Roar: Facing Conflict and Transforming Defensiveness into Healthy Aggression

"In response to threat and injury, animals, including humans, execute biologically based, non-conscious action patterns that prepare them to meet the threat and defend themselves..."
Peter A. Levine[12]

I hated being called a goody two shoes. That used to really piss me off. Of course, I'd never tell you that to your face, but if you have the gall to blame me for something I didn't do or treat me

---

12   Ideas as presented in: Levine, Peter A. *Waking the Tiger: Healing Trauma: The Innate Capacity to Transform Overwhelming Experiences.* North Atlantic Books, 1997

like I did something "bad," watch out. This "Good Girl" might just give you a glimpse of all she is repressing. I know how to get angry and stand up for myself. If you accuse me of something that goes against my values, the advocate in me will rear her ugly head.

She came out in full swing at a 7-Eleven gas station one Saturday morning when I was about twelve or thirteen. My friend and I had walked (or more likely turned cartwheels) up the street to get a snack, counting how many it took to get there, like the licks to get to the center of a tootsie roll pop. We'd been looking through the candy aisle trying to decide what we wanted, which is a tough decision for any kid, when I finally selected a Hershey's bar, imagining how good it would taste to lick off the wrapper after sitting it in the sun at the pool later that day. I walked up and down the aisle, waiting for my friend to make her decision, and at the last minute, changed my mind. I'm allowed to do that, right? I can't remember exactly what I saw that beckoned me instead, but I put the Hershey bar back and traded it for something more tantalizing.

When I laid it on the counter and got ready to pay, the lady at the cash register looked at me with accusing eyes and said, "Where is the other candy bar you picked up?"

"I put it back," I replied. She didn't believe me and demanded I show her what was in my pockets. Drum roll. Picture the little girl who made an unconscious decision a long time ago to always be good, and imagine how that false accusation might land. All bets were off. She already thought of me as bad, so there was nothing to lose, right? The risk was gone, and I no longer had any reason to be polite, so out roared my anger, setting her straight and letting her know it was not okay to treat me that way. I can't recall the exact words I used, but I clearly remember the energy I felt in my chest when I ripped off my coat and flung it on the counter. It was something like, "If you don't believe me, check my pockets yourself! I did not steal anything!" It still feels good just thinking about it. Maybe it was a little more aggressive than the incident called for, but I'm pretty sure that energy was connected to some past offenses where I'd felt less emboldened to set the record straight.

I didn't know this lady from Adam, so I didn't care about protecting my relationship with her. She didn't scare me, nor did I have reason to respect her, which allowed me the freedom to defend myself and say what I wanted to say. I walked out of there a little taller that day. There was a confidence I was carrying home with me that felt like maybe I had gotten out of the store with something that I didn't pay for. The lesson: don't ever accuse a "Good Girl" of being bad, especially when you don't have all the facts.

The Fight Response

The part of me that got mad that day is the same part that works tirelessly to ensure I'm seen in a good light. It's my inner defense attorney, shouting: *Don't you know how hard I work to do everything right? How dare you accuse me of something I didn't do.* The injustice of her accusation that day in the 7-Eleven activated something primal in me—a fierce need to defend my integrity unleashed the roar of my fight response. Most of us don't access that side of ourselves so easily, especially in our closest relationships. When the stakes are high and approval feels vital, we're more likely to suppress that energy, internalize accusations, and stew in resentment. I know because I've done that, too.

For years, I struggled to navigate conflicts without crumbling in the face of others' confidence. Early in my marriage, my husband and I had countless arguments that left me feeling crushed. His certainty and strong presence often made me question my own perspective. Anytime he misunderstood my intentions, I would think: *Can't you see my heart? I would never pick a fight or hurt you intentionally.* Being seen as the source of conflict felt like a slap in the face and a betrayal of my core values. It was disorienting, and worse, it made me start questioning how others perceived me—and even how I saw myself.

It wasn't until I learned to shift out of reaction mode and channel that defensive energy into clear, courageous communication and life direction that things began to change. I realized my fight response wasn't something to be suppressed but harnessed. It was the energy my body was giving me to create change. The key was learning how to channel it into healthy aggression—a force that drives positive, transformative action. I'll never forget the day my eight-year-old daughter modeled that for me during an Upward Basketball Game.

Getting in Touch with Our Power

I sat on the bleachers with the other moms and watched in horror as my little girl wrestled the basketball away from a girl on the opposing team, knocking her down in her fight for possession. I should have been cheering, but instead, I shrank down in embarrassment, thinking, *Where did my sweet girl go, and what have you taught her?*

She had always been a little too polite on the court for my husband's liking. Apparently, he'd spent the last practice teaching the girls how to get aggressive and steal the ball. That day, my daughter saw her opportunity, reached in, grabbed the ball, and won a chance to dribble it down the court and shoot. She walked off the court afterward, her disheveled ponytail a badge of honor, reflecting her newfound grit and determination.

Assertiveness is not incompatible with kindness. It's the embodiment of our God-given power. Love doesn't stand around hoping for a chance to take a shot. It's the force that creates things! When we ground ourselves in that power, we have the capacity to shift the energy in a room. That's the same force we need to harness, not just to win basketball games but to reclaim our health, transform our relationships, and move toward our goals and dreams.

From Passivity to Power

This lesson came to life again while babysitting my son's dog, Venice. She was dominating my golden retriever, Honey, taking over her toys and territory. At first, Honey responded with passivity, retreating, and letting Venice have her way. But something shifted on day two. Honey found her bark, growling and standing her ground. From that moment on, the dynamic between the dogs transformed. They played together with mutual respect, no longer driven by dominance or submission.

The same principle applies to us. When we suppress our fight energy, we lose confidence and safety in our own space. But when we access healthy aggression, we reclaim our ability to advocate for ourselves and create balance in our relationships.

Channeling Fight Energy into Transformation

I saw this power at work with a client recently. She had been feeling powerless, afraid she was never going to overcome her anxiety and depression. During her first session, she shared that she wanted healthier relationships, to feel more confident and less fearful of rejection. She wanted to stop feeling so guilty and angry when she tried to say *No* to her mother and sisters, who were more outspoken and dominant than her. She felt like she always had to be guarded, unable to trust them, and rated her average stress level an 8/10. When I asked what the costs of nothing changing were, she acknowledged, "Continued loneliness, health problems, and having to up my meds or check myself into a mental hospital."

Her biggest obstacle to lowering her stress and not shutting down in depression was not being able to speak up for herself.

She stated, "I want to be able to say what I want to say without screaming. Why can't I express myself?"

We did a somatic (body-based) exercise designed to get in touch with her healthy aggression so she could speak with confidence in a conversation she needed to have with her sister regarding her parent's care. She knew she needed to make some changes and create some boundaries for her own well-being, but guilt and fear were holding her back while resentment built, causing a rift between her and her sisters.

During the exercise, I asked her to press her palm against mine and apply force while I met and matched her energy. As she did, she began to feel the strength and power she held to shift things. In just three minutes, she went from feeling powerless to feeling filled with hope and possibility. Later, she texted me: "I had a really good conversation with my sister today! Thanks for your help." Her results speak to the importance of restoring our sense of power as a prescription for our chronic emotional and physical health conditions.

Harnessing Healthy Aggression

When we hear the word "aggression," we often picture fighting, bullying, or someone overpowering another, like a dog baring its teeth. However, aggression is also the force necessary for breakthroughs. Just like words, money, or influence, aggression is a neutral energy that can be used for good or evil. When it's rooted in insecurity and powerlessness, it drives reactive, defensive, destructive, and self-sabotaging behaviors, but when it's grounded in love and confidence, aggression becomes a constructive force.

I saw this dichotomy play out when my son played defensive end in high school. His primary job was to get around the offensive line and take out the quarterback. We watched from the stands as he raised up on his cleats, shifted his weight over clenched, tape-covered fists, and primed his strength to explode into action when the ball was hiked. The fans stood and roared with us when he came around from behind, wrapped his arms around the QB, and took him to the ground before the play had a chance of being executed. The goal was not to harm but to use his strength to outmaneuver his opponent, and when done with skill, the outcome was respected. The QB, though deflated and frustrated, often gave him a head nod, acknowledging the fair play and my son would receive it without any hard feelings either way. The energy of the moment coursed through him as he rejoined his teammates, igniting a ripple of determination down the line.

This natural flow of assertive energy contrasts sharply with what we, as women, are often taught. Unlike other mammals, we've been conditioned to contain our natural aggression, suppress our instincts, and act civilized. We've been told: *Don't show off. Don't act puffed up. Make sure not to make the other team feel bad. Restrain yourself.*

The problem with this conditioning is that, in our efforts to appear appropriate, humble, and polite, we end up putting a choke collar around our God-given power. We're so afraid of our power that we'd rather hold ourselves back, hinder, and defer it, sabotaging the impact and fruitfulness designed to ripple out from it.

There were also times I witnessed my son's frustration build with missed tackles, bad calls, and exhaustion, leading him to take it out on another player and earn a penalty flag. Instead of standing and cheering, our bodies contracted on the benches, willing him to pull back. Our experiences of unhealthy aggression cause many of us to swing to the opposite extreme, vowing a life of humility to avoid being perceived as cocky or trying to steal God's glory. We even justify our shrinking back, quoting scriptures like Romans 12:3 to remind us not to think more highly of ourselves than we ought.

However, it's crucial to distinguish between true humility and fear-driven passivity. True humility involves an honest recognition of our strengths and weaknesses, using our power responsibly and without arrogance. It is rooted in love and confidence, enabling us to step forward boldly with a healthy interdependency on God and others. In contrast, shrinking back and suppressing our power can be just as harmful as misusing it. Both responses stem from fear, but it's the fear that destroys—not the natural energy of aggression. True humility doesn't require denying our God-given power or avoiding assertiveness. Instead, it invites us to channel our healthy aggression with courage and purpose, stepping into our role as empowered individuals ready to make a meaningful impact. Yet, for many of us, this balance feels elusive. The line between asserting ourselves and staying in other's good graces can feel like a tightrope we're always tip-toeing on. This tension was all too familiar to me, as I discovered one morning when a vivid dream brought buried emotions to the surface.

Balancing Assertiveness and Approval

I woke up one morning with a familiar and unwelcome feeling in my body—like I was in trouble, being judged, or someone was unhappy with me. Alongside this feeling, anger began rising up, as if to say, *How dare you assert your power over me? You don't get to control me, shame me, or take away my freedom. I need to feel safe as I go through my day without worrying about you judging my every action.*

In my dream, I was standing at a mirror, putting on makeup in what seemed to be my old work office. Out of the corner of my eye, I caught sight of my former boss watching me. Something shifted inside me, and I began frantically trying to finish, fumbling to get my makeup brush and eyeshadow back into the case, like a child afraid of being caught and reprimanded. When I woke up, I felt like I'd been transported back in time—not just to that workplace but to that ten-year-old girl that vowed to never do anything that gave others an opportunity to think badly about her.

My boss was someone who rarely offered validation or feedback to confirm she valued my contributions. While I respected her, I often felt scrutinized and found myself walking on eggshells around her, careful not to do anything that might give her reason to question me. I'd witnessed how abruptly she'd let my fellow co-workers go when they challenged her philosophy. That internal battle—between maintaining her approval and moving through the clinic authentically—felt like a tightrope I was constantly walking.

I always felt like she was watching over my shoulder, ensuring I was doing things the way she would, and it wasn't a pleasant feeling for me. I had always won people over easily—colleagues and clients usually liked me, thought highly of me, and often told me how much they appreciated my work or what a good therapist I was. But not her. In one breath, she'd tell me I had freedom over my schedule; in the next, she'd hold control over it or express frustration if I made adjustments without her permission.

From Sensitive to Secure: The Sting of Criticism

I don't know what triggered my dream that night, but it reflected a familiar inner struggle—the tension between seeking approval and moving freely in my autonomy. At work, I thrived when left to my own devices, responding confidently to patients' needs, researching to expand my skills, and trusting my instincts. But as soon as I felt scrutinized—whether by my boss second-guessing me or my husband hovering in the kitchen—I froze. The criticism, even unspoken, felt personal, undermining my confidence and stirring up resentment.

Hovering behaviors and micromanagement erode trust and stifle growth, not just in the workplace but in relationships. Criticism is a really crappy motivator. It pushes us into defensive patterns—either withdrawing or overcompensating to prove our worth. When our self-worth hinges on external validation, criticism feels like rejection, a painful echo of past wounds.

But the sting of criticism is also an opportunity. It invites us to pause, reflect, and remind ourselves of the truth: *Our worth is not tied to what we do.* By separating our identity from our work, we create the internal safety needed to accept feedback and grow. We make space to learn, make mistakes, and move toward fulfillment.

Separating Our Identity From What We Do

Many service-driven women over-identify with what they do for others, making it difficult not to take criticism personally. We learn to help others to feel validated, loved, and needed—but when that validation is withheld, it feels like rejection. This can lead to spirals of anxiety: *What did I do wrong? Why don't they want what I have to offer?*

To escape this cycle, we have to untangle our identity from the value of what we do. When we approach our work from a secure, self-led place, we stop looking to others to fill the gaps in our sense of worth. We can ask for and receive feedback with curiosity instead of defensiveness, focusing on growth instead of self-preservation.

This shift is about reclaiming our strength and confidence. It's not just about feeling more at ease—it's about pushing past fear, setting boundaries, and moving toward our full potential. Healthy aggression plays a critical role here, empowering us to show up authentically and advocate for ourselves with courage and clarity.

Moving Beyond Defensiveness and Embracing Responsibility

One of the ways I've learned to move beyond defensiveness is through honest and courageous communication. For example, I've said, "Hey, I appreciate your attention to detail and how much you value things being done a certain way, but I feel scrutinized when you watch and correct me as I work. It feeds my insecurity, causing me to make more mistakes. I'd love it if you'd give me the space to learn and make mistakes my own way. I'm working on building self-trust, and your support would mean a lot. The more confident I feel, the more open I'll be to feedback without feeling defensive. I value the way your eye for detail helps keep things running smoothly, and I appreciate your understanding."

This kind of communication allows me to articulate my needs without blame or defensiveness. It helps me stand confidently and avoid making others' words or actions define me. I've learned I don't need to take things personally or get defensive; instead, I can remain neutral, secure in myself, and approach others with understanding.

This lesson has also transformed how I approach feedback in my work as a coach. A business coach once helped me identify my need for feedback to evaluate whether my clients were making progress and achieving their goals. I realized that having systems for gathering feedback wasn't just about improving my services; it was also about creating a foundation of trust and communication. Now, I conduct pre- and post-session check-ins and send periodic feedback forms, giving clients a safe space to share what they appreciate, what they'd like more of, and what needs adjustment. Including this process in client agreements signals how much I value honest communication and helps me serve them at the highest level. On days when I feel uncertain, I can revisit this feedback to remind myself of the positive impact I'm making.

By separating the value of my services from my personal worth, I've learned to approach feedback with curiosity and confidence, using it as a tool for growth rather than a measure of my identity. This shift not only helps me as a coach but also sets an example for my clients, encouraging them to embrace honest communication in their own lives.

A Force for Change

Healthy aggression is the energy our body gives us to create change. It says, "This is enough. Step back. That's not okay." It's the voice that stands strong in the face of fear, speaks up with conviction, and acts with integrity. This energy isn't destructive or domineering—it's constructive. It channels our courage and autonomy into setting boundaries, pursuing goals, and stepping into our power.

The fight response is wired into us for a reason. It says, "Not on my watch," when something crosses the line. It moves into action when a child reaches for something dangerous and declares a strong *No!* when someone makes unwanted advances. It matches the energy of the bully without sinking to their level. It is secure enough to turn the other cheek, but it does not cower. It moves out of its comfort zone with courage, overcoming the chains of the past, and walks into the growth zone with its head high and chest expanded, unafraid to take up space.

Begin by noticing how your fight response currently shows up. Are you suppressing it, reacting defensively, or harnessing it constructively? Approach these habits with compassion. Remember, they were once protective mechanisms. They just need to know you've grown—ready and able to stand in your power. With each moment of courageous action, those inner critics and people pleasers can step back, trusting you to lead.

Here are some signs that you might be repressing healthy aggression.

- Feelings of powerlessness
- Frequent passive-aggressive behaviors: indirect expression of anger or frustration through silence or sarcasm
- Avoiding conflict or confrontation
- Chronic People-Pleasing: Consistently prioritizing others' needs over your own, often at your own expense
- False Humility: Downplaying your achievements or abilities to avoid standing out or making others uncomfortable
- Difficulty Saying No: Agreeing to requests or demands even when it causes you stress or over-commitment
- Suppressed Anger: Feeling irritable or resentful but not expressing it, leading to internalized stress

Signs that you are harnessing healthy aggression include:

- Setting clear boundaries and feeling comfortable enforcing them
- Standing up for yourself with calm assertiveness
- Advocating for your needs and desires with confidence
- Facing challenges head-on with courage and resilience
- Expressing your feelings openly and honestly
- Moving toward goals despite fear or uncertainty

Noticing these patterns is the first step to unlocking the power to create meaningful change. Imagine the ripple effect that would have on your life and those around you!

GOOD GIRL RX: Harness Your Fight Response for Positive Change

Your fight response is a powerful ally, not an enemy. By learning to recognize and work with this energy, you can reclaim your voice, assert your needs, and create meaningful change in your life. Transformation begins when you stop fearing this energy and start using it as a force for good.

Reflection Questions:

1. How does your fight response show up? Think about a recent time when you felt criticized or misunderstood. How did you react? What emotions or physical sensations arose in your body?
2. What makes you angry? Are there common situations or relationships that activate your fight response? What might that anger be trying to protect and defend?
3. Reflect on a time you felt defensive in a relationship. What beliefs or fears were fueling your reaction? What were the stories arising? How might you use the energy of your fight response to communicate your needs and desires with courage?
4. The next time you feel anger or defensiveness arise, what small action could you take to address the situation with authenticity and integrity?

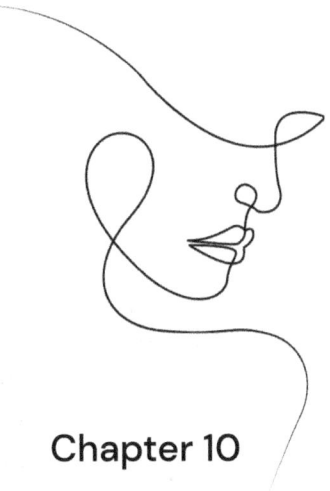

Chapter 10

Conditioned to Fawn: Unpacking Habits of Pleasing and Appeasing

> *"Our nervous system's need for safety can lead to patterns of appeasement that serve to protect us in the short term but trap us in a cycle of self-abandonment."*
> Irene Lyon[13]

Ann's Story

As a young girl, Ann was taught that her role was to serve others: "I grew up learning what I needed to know to become a housewife and was told, *'That's what we do as women.'* The idea of disappointing anyone by not being what they envisioned for me wasn't even something I considered. I didn't even think about what I wanted. I didn't know I had other options." Ann

---

[13] Lyon, Irene. SAFETY: A Nervous System & Somatic Perspective. 21 Apr. 2024, irenelyon.com

continued, "My aunt shared a funny memory with me from when I was a little girl. I was misbehaving in some way, and my parents told me to be good, and I replied, '*I don't want to be good; I want to be happy!*' I'd been a little rebel until I was five, but after that, I became perfect, always getting good grades, doing what I was supposed to, never getting in trouble. I was homeschooled, which involved day in and day out learning. If I complained about doing my math or science, my mom would say, '*Life is not always fun.*'"

"Now I have a hard time stepping out of experiences I don't want to be in and get in abusive and unwanted situations," Anne told me with a sad sigh. "Knowing what I want and being able to dream and step into it is hard for me. It seems almost impossible sometimes. I have such a fear of disappointing people."

In her adult life, this pattern persisted, shaping her relationships and leading to an abusive five-year marriage that not only eroded her sense of self but also took a toll on her physical and emotional well-being. "I started having chronic migraines, and a year in, I was diagnosed with an autoimmune disease. When I finally got the courage to leave my ex, I experienced panic attacks. I realized I struggled with anxiety before that, but it took a long time for me to recognize it. Ann's challenges extended into her professional life. She found herself in a toxic work environment with a narcissistic boss and a co-worker who sexually harassed her. Despite recognizing the need to leave, she felt guilty about the impact her departure might have on her elderly boss. She admits,"Others have quit, but I feel bad for people. Wanting to make everyone happy hurts me professionally."

The Fawn Response

Ann's experience highlights a survival pattern known as the fawn response. Therapist Pete Walker, who coined the term, describes fawning as "a response to a threat by becoming more appealing to the threat," often through pleasing or appeasing behaviors to diffuse conflict and feel safe.[14]

Common Signs of Fawning
- Saying "yes" when every part of you wants to say "no."
- Feeling anxious when someone is upset with you.
- Apologizing for things that aren't your fault.
- Deprioritizing your needs to focus on others' comfort.
- Silencing your opinions to keep the peace.

For women like Ann, fawning isn't a conscious choice—it's a conditioned response. When our autonomy and individuation are reflected to us as selfish and wrong, children have no other choice but to self-abandon for the sake of attachment. To survive, girls learn to restrain their natural impulses, suppress their voices, and yield their will to please others. But the cost is steep: they don't just become compliant; they become easy prey for predators. Instead of *"run, fight back, or get away!"* their internal protector whispers, *"Be quiet. Don't scream. Don't be seen as defiant. This is how you stay safe."*

What begins as a survival mechanism soon becomes a trap—like tying a dog's leash to a post to keep it protected, only to find it twisted and unable to reach its water bowl. What was meant to keep us safe ends up harming us.

Girls born with more sensitivity don't even need to be spanked to curb their sense of agency and expression–all it takes is a look of disapproval, a tone of displeasure, or a lack of attunement. Those fortunate enough to have a stronger will to begin with, those we can not seem to "tame"–well, they become the "bad" girls, labeled and shamed as the black sheep of the family. But here's the hard truth: while one may face societal

---

14 Walker, Pete. *Complex PTSD: From Surviving to Thriving—A Guide and Map for Recovering from Childhood Trauma.* CreateSpace Independent Publishing Platform, 2013.

rejection, the other is left vulnerable to abuse. Who is truly safe in this dynamic?

The Hidden Cost of Fawning

The fawn response leads to pervasive patterns of self-abandonment that take a heavy toll on women's health and well-being. Shutting down our life force for the sake of attachment may protect us from being seen as rude and rebellious, but it sends a powerful message to our brains that it's not safe to release our inhibitions and move freely in the world. We may survive, but thriving requires the safety to step into self-leadership and take courageous action. It requires an update in the narratives your body holds that say happiness and fun are wrong and selfish.

These learned survival habits are the number one thing holding us back and keeping us sick, stuck, or caught in endless loops of repeating challenges and relational dynamics. In order to help my clients move through resistance, I had to learn more about why they weren't feeling safe. I knew through my training that if someone wasn't experiencing the outcome they wanted, something must feel at risk. I understood this cognitively, but it wasn't until I witnessed it that I began to understand just how much our body memories affect our adult experiences.

Disarmed: Laura's Story

I got a call from a client one day who was trying to recover from a recent hip surgery. Instead of being able to rest, heal, and use the time to step back from obligations, she felt really, really scared and helpless. She scheduled an appointment to get a prescription for antidepressants.

I led her through an exercise to help her get some distance from the insecurity she was feeling and explore what she needed to feel safe enough to rest. I stood with her, five feet away from the chair, facing the fear she'd left sitting there, and listened as she got curious and gave it a voice. From that distance, she found her own personalized prescription: things like being outside, creative pursuits, and being surrounded by the safe, supportive people in her life. She landed intuitively on the resources her nervous system needed to calm her body's alarms and restore her sense of safety so she could relax and heal.

The depression was a byproduct of the shame that was coming up in her vulnerability. She wasn't able to use her fawn response or please anyone from her sick bed. This left her feeling exposed and stripped of her defenses. When we can't do the things we need to feel secure, the only option is to shut down and immobilize ourselves in a freeze response, just like a mammal in the wild might do. A white-tailed fawn knows to watch for predators before running and leaping in the meadow. If it senses danger, it gets quiet and watchful, just like little Laura did instinctively. Imagine how helpless and exposed that fawn might feel if it was lying in the middle of the field with an injury to its hip. Can you feel the anxiety? The terror? That is what Laura was feeling after her surgery. She couldn't run away, fight back, or appease anyone, leaving her defenseless. Her body was doing the only other thing it could do: curl into a fetal position (only I'm guessing that was difficult with her hip in a brace). Can you feel the vulnerability of that? The darkness? I believe it's the same darkness Jesus experienced hanging from the cross–the same sense of disconnection and abandonment. That's what trauma does. It leaves us feeling separated from our resources and unable to see the light of hope. No wonder Laura wanted antidepressants.

Her depression was a last resort of her brilliant biological design, not a sign she was broken. Her body was just detecting danger and trying to keep her alive. That shut-down helps numb the pain and terror and disconnect us from it, the same way a rabbit being held in the mouth of a predator might need to do.

Laura had shared her history of early sexual abuse, which she'd gone through counseling for as an adult. She had talked through it but had never worked with the body and the alarms still living within it. She had signed up for coaching support to work on developing healthier habits of self-care and stronger boundaries, areas that were challenging for her to prioritize. She knew if she could have some regular rhythms and do less, she'd feel more of the peace and the presence of God that she longed for. She'd been trying everything from supplements, hormone replacement, nutrition, prayer, and Bible study to get that peace. She struggled with chronic anxiety, ADHD, overwhelm, and exhaustion. She had been diagnosed with fibromyalgia and Hashimoto's Thyroiditis, an autoimmune condition. More recently, she'd been having recurring hip pain that wasn't getting better and had opted for surgery to repair a tendon.

In our work together, Laura shared that her dad had used a reward chart to encourage "pleasing behaviors" and how much she worked for that praise. She had a strong fear of abandonment and hated disappointing people. In previous sessions, we'd bumped up against a lot of resistance when she tried to implement action steps to support her body's healing and her soul's need for joy and fulfillment. She struggled to make time to swim at the YMCA, a practice that was incredibly regulating to her nervous system and allowed her body to feel safe and relaxed. She'd set timers to go off to remind her to stop what she was doing and draw herself a bath, but couldn't make herself stop what she was doing, always feeling pulled toward what she "should" be doing instead.

When working through the resistance one session, we traced her felt sense of restlessness and anxiety in her body back to an early memory of her two-year-old self at the home daycare she went to, standing at a wall, tuned into her environment, eyes and ears scanning for danger instead of playing like the other kids. Her body was programmed to be on guard and protect her from vulnerability. Pleasing, fawning, over responding, saying yes, and avoiding relaxation and play was a conditioned habit that had kept her alive and safe. The fawn response kept her mobilized, responding to other's needs, saying yes to things she later regretted, leaving her in a constant state of overwhelm and anxiety. It kept her going until her stress capacity reached its window of tolerance, and she got sick. Her body shut down in an effort to conserve energy.

How the Fawn Response Impacts Our Bodies

Biology of Trauma expert Dr. Amy Apigan states, "If there is a trauma response there are going to be health challenges. The trauma response changes the operating system of our body. It is a biological response. It changes everything down to the tissue level, organ level, DNA level."[15]

Research is increasingly highlighting the profound link between stress and health. Studies, such as those conducted by Felitti et al. (1998), reveal how Adverse Childhood Experiences (ACEs) can lead to lasting impacts on physical and mental health, emphasizing that early trauma significantly shapes the body's stress response system.[16] Dr. Apigan and other practitioners describe this as "trauma physiology," a state where the body shifts from a typical stress response to a trauma response when its capacity to cope is overwhelmed. Overwhelm is often seen as purely emotional, but it is deeply physiological. It reflects the body's way of saying, *"That is too much, too fast, or too little for*

---

15   Apigian, Aimie. *"The Biology of Attachment, Survival, and Resilience."* Trauma Healing Accelerated, 2025, https://traumahealingaccelerated.com/biology-of-attachment-survival-and-resilience-adv/.

16   Felitti, Vincent J., et al. "Relationship of Childhood Abuse and Household Dysfunction to Many of the Leading Causes of Death in Adults: The Adverse Childhood Experiences (ACE) Study." *American Journal of Preventive Medicine*, vol. 14, no. 4, 1998, pp. 245–258. doi:10.1016/S0749-3797(98)00017-8.

too long." This aligns with the definition of trauma as anything that overwhelms the body's capacity and resources, leading to shutdown and setting the stage for chronic illness, pain, and disease. Biological responses such as hormonal, endocrine, and neurochemical changes, along with increased inflammatory markers, reveal how trauma impacts our systems. As Bessel van der Kolk (2014) emphasizes, *the body keeps the score*, encoding these trauma responses into our very biology.[17]

While hormonal, endocrine, and neurochemical changes, as well as inflammatory markers, are observable in our biology, they are ultimately manifestations of our deep-seated survival drives. If we address our biology without addressing our safety programming, we will stay stuck in a loop of chronic health challenges, longing to feel good again but never feeling safe enough to allow it.

Chronic fawning adds another layer of harm. When your worth is tied to your usefulness, your personal boundaries, identity, and self-esteem begin to erode. This constant self-abandonment blocks self-care and prevents the formation of genuinely supportive relationships. Focusing on pleasing others leaves little room for mutual satisfaction or authentic connection, creating persistent distress. Over time, this chronic stress and vigilance reduces the body's natural resilience and starts manifesting as health issues.

Research by Klimek et al. (2018) highlights that adverse experiences lower resiliency and heighten vulnerability to both physical and mental illnesses.[18] Similarly, Felitti et al. (1998) found that individuals with higher ACE scores, which often

---

17 van der Kolk, Bessel A. *The Body Keeps the Score: Brain, Mind, and Body in the Healing of Trauma.* Viking, 2014.
18 Klimek, Peter, et al. "The Impact of Adverse Childhood Experiences on Health in Early and Later Life: A Systematic Review of Meta-Analyses." *Epidemiology and Psychiatric Sciences*, vol. 29, no. e82, 2018, pp. 1–10. doi:10.1017/S2045796018000633.

correlate with chronic fawning behaviors, have a dysregulated nervous system, predisposing them to a range of chronic health conditions, including:

- Asthma
- Depression
- Fibromyalgia
- Headaches
- Allergies
- Diabetes
- Anxiety
- Gastrointestinal problems
- High blood pressure
- Rheumatoid arthritis
- Cancer[19]

Understanding the impact of the fawn response on physical and emotional health is crucial for healing. By recognizing the deep-seated patterns that drive fawning behavior, women can begin to reclaim their boundaries, rebuild their self-esteem, and develop healthier, more reciprocal relationships. Healing from the fawn response involves not only addressing the psychological wounds but also nurturing the body and nervous system back to a state of balance and resilience.

What Fawning Looks Like in Action

Fawning is a conditioned response where our first impulse is to make others feel good about themselves, meet their needs, and make sure they're happy as a way to avoid the anxiety we feel when they're not. We become highly thought of, but we stay hidden, hurting, unknown, and alone. As hard as we try, we can't

---

19 Felitti et al., "The Adverse Childhood Experiences (ACE) Study," 1998.

figure out how to make ourselves seen because this strategy is blocking our authenticity.

When I was researching the word "dutiful" for the previous chapter, I was struck by one of the synonyms listed under the definition: "fawning," as in the fawn response. Being the word nerd that I am, I had to keep digging and was rewarded with a new word to add to my vocabulary bank: "obsequious," meaning too eager to help or obey someone important. That is exactly what fawning is–an over-eagerness that turns into people-pleasing and appeasing behaviors.

These synonyms provide a clear picture of what the fawn response looks like in action: "obliging, agreeable, restrained, meek, yielding, constrained, disciplined, submissive, inhibited, and repressed." When we've been told that being quiet and toned down is appropriate behavior for a woman, fawning becomes an efficient strategy to ensure we are viewed as good. We're told this is what it looks like to be graceful, tasteful, and modest; what is becoming of a woman. Passages like 1 Timothy 2:9, where Paul emphasizes modesty and godliness, have often been interpreted as instructions for women to avoid drawing attention to themselves. While the text calls for humility, cultural interpretations have sometimes extended this into expectations that women should be unnoticeable and silent. Many church leaders interpret these teachings as a mandate for women to be subdued and quiet in the pews. This is how a "good" woman behaves. So we comply, and we fawn. After all, who wants to be thought of as tasteless, graceless, and loud?

Protected From Displeasure

It doesn't take a big trauma for women to have fawning as their default operating system. The real trauma is not what happens to us but the automatic repression of self-will in the midst of what is happening to us—the self-abandonment required for us to feel safe.

While fawning is often a necessary and very appropriate survival response to stay alive in situations of abuse, this learned habit can handicap a woman's ability to express herself and take confident action. It becomes a choke collar, inhibiting not only her expression but her ability to roll in the grass, leap, dance, and move in sweet abandon because her body equates freedom with rebellion and danger. It doesn't feel safe to question your mother and father, your pastor, or what you've been taught as the inherent Word of God. Stepping outside the 'umbrella of protection' can feel as terrifying as when Rapunzel first considered leaving the tower—her mother's warnings echoing that staying was for her own good. No wonder she experienced internal torment as she considered the freedom her soul was calling out for. The risk felt huge. Everything in her said, *"Don't go that way. It's not safe to think that, entertain that, or dip your toe in that water. Something really bad could happen."* When our bodies hold the narrative that to question is to risk the unpardonable sin and eternal separation, our nervous system sees our attempts to break free as life-threatening.

Bernie Seigel, M.D., and author of the book *Love, Medicine and Miracles: Lessons Learned about Self-Healing from a Surgeon's Experience with Exceptional Patients*, explains this resistance well: "Old patterns, though painful, are easier. Change is difficult, uncomfortable and frightening."[20]

Surviving to Thriving

Laura is still working on her boundaries, communicating her needs, and pausing to interrupt her compulsion to say yes to

---

20 Siegel, Bernie S. *Love, Medicine & Miracles: Lessons Learned about Self-Healing from a Surgeon's Experience with Exceptional Patients*. Harper & Row, 1986.

people. Although she still experiences some weeks where she feels overwhelmed and becomes ill, she has made significant progress. She now has a more profound compassion and understanding for herself, leading to better overall health, more quality time with her family, and increased confidence as she explores her interests and takes action to prioritize them. She's currently pain-free and was able to complete a two-year Transformational Ministries Program this year. That's huge when you feel like you never finish what you start because you can't prioritize your own goals and desires! She wept tears at her graduation and shared, "It's so important for me to see myself set a goal and follow through. I did it!"

Those celebrations are so important when your life has been driven by an underlying fear that God will walk away from you if you don't do enough to please Him. It's not enough to go to church, read the Bible, and pray if our bodies are feeling disconnected because of the state of our nervous system. So many women assume if they can't feel God's peace and presence, they must be doing something wrong. This is not about right or wrong behavior. It's about self-preservation, and it doesn't help to have someone tell you that you just need to surrender and go all in. That advice, although well meaning, can often perpetuate the very survival states we need to break free from for healing. We'd never tell that little girl standing with her back to the wall, paralyzed in fear, that she just needs to put on the whole armor of God and renew her mind. You would never tell her she just needs to read her Bible, declare more affirmations, and resist the devil. I hope you would say, "I'm so sorry you aren't feeling safe. What can I do to help you feel more secure?"

Maybe her answer would be similar to Laura's when she realized she had overcommitted again and was avoiding her phone, worried if she answered it she'd take on something and extend energy she didn't have to give. *"I hear that you are nervous. Let me hold you until you don't feel scared anymore."*

GOOD GIRL RX: Cultivate Safety & Reassurance From Within

Our bodies are hardwired to keep us safe, responding in ways that once served us but can now keep us from experiencing true connection and confidence. This chapter is an invitation to gently explore how these patterns may be impacting your well-being. By examining your story with compassion, you can begin to break free from automatic responses and create space for a more empowered, authentic self.

Reflection Questions:

1. Reflect on the experiences shared by Ann and Laura in this chapter. What parts of their stories resonated with you or felt familiar? What insights or takeaways emerged for you as you read? Take some time to journal your thoughts, noticing any parallels to your own experiences and the lessons you're beginning to uncover about your own fawn response.
2. Think of a time when you felt calm, secure, or supported. What were the people, places, or actions that helped you feel safe? How can you bring more of these resources into your daily life when you feel triggered to please or self-abandon?
3. If you could offer reassurance to a part of yourself that learned to please and adapt to feel safe, what would you say? If that feels challenging, what would you say to someone else having this same experience? How can you extend that same compassion to yourself?

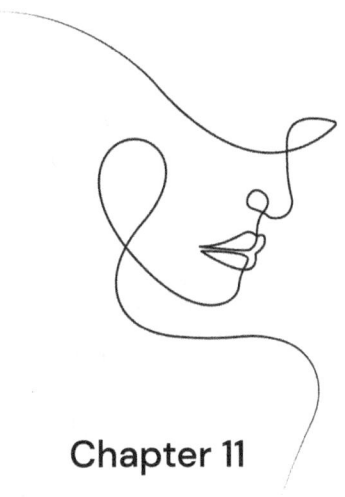

Chapter 11

Paralyzed by Fear: Understanding Her Freeze Response

"Safety is not the absence of threat; it is the presence of connection. Healing begins when we align with our internal resources and recognize that we are no longer helpless."
Gabor Mate

I used to dread being home alone. If I heard a noise, I'd scan for the source but never go looking for it. That was crazy talk. Who does that? I'd sit through movies where the actors did that and be like, *Stop! What are you nuts? That's how you get killed!*

I can still remember that feeling of paralysis as I froze and kept my body really, really still. My muscle fibers tensed like springs, loaded and ready to burst into a run or throw a punch if needed. You can't relax, and your mind is going ninety to nothing to listen, detect, be alert—planning and scheming, thinking of all the options to get away if someone comes through the door.

It wasn't until I was married that I finally learned how to overcome this and feel safe in my own home. One night, when my husband was traveling, I got tired of lying there, paralyzed by fear, and decided to get my power back. I visualized myself standing up to the threat and defeating it as I rehearsed my script and practiced what I would say. I didn't wait passively for them to come into my room but got up and met them at the door. I stood in my power and told them off—of course, in *'good girl' talk*. I declared, *I'm not afraid of you, and I will no longer let you bully me or rob me of my sleep. You can take my life if you want, but you will not take my confidence and steal my peace anymore.*

I laid there reminding myself that if God wanted to, He could blind them and keep me hidden, and it was safe to sleep and allow myself to be protected by the armies of heaven that were fully capable of surrounding me. I told myself that He could just as easily protect me from feeling any pain and whisk me away into His presence or hold me in the safety of His arms if someone should try to attack me. As I lay there rehearsing it all, the fear that had held me in bondage left my body, and I fell into a deep, peaceful sleep with a smile on my face, proud of how I stood up and defeated the enemy.

I had no idea what I was doing at the time or why this worked so well. I was taught all my life to trust in God, have faith, and that He could protect me, but I didn't realize I needed to align with His power within me to activate that. It wasn't just about trusting a source outside of myself and lying there passively, hoping that He would slay the giants. Instead, I realized the giant that needed slaying wasn't at my door—it was stored in my body memories. That fear was born long before the night my husband left on a work trip. It was merely triggered by the sounds I heard—sounds that my nervous system recognized as echoes of a time when those very noises were frightening and overwhelming. A time when I lacked the resources and comfort to feel safe, when no one was there to reassure me or guide me back to a place of confidence. I didn't realize that overcoming that *"freeze"* response required me to complete *the story* and bring it to a resolution so I could move from helplessness to empowered again. I had to actually allow my body to discharge that energy that was compressed, like releasing a rubber band you've pulled back. My body needed that to happen to get the message that I was safe by going through the story the way it should have gone down.

In his book, *Walking the Tiger*, trauma expert Peter Levine explains this immobility response and how the experiences where we've felt threatened or overwhelmed can lead to us becoming physiologically stuck in this *freeze* response.[21] Our body learns to *"resign"* itself to a state where the act of escaping does not exist. This resigned behavior or paralysis is the same survival strategy seen in animal behavior. If you have ever seen a possum play dead or an impala go limp when being attacked, you've witnessed this natural, God-designed self-preservation strategy. Unfortunately, unless and until we shake the trauma off or release it from the body and *"primitive brain,"* we remain stuck, to varying degrees, in a traumatized state. In order to move and take action with confidence, we have to create a new experience where we actively escape so the body can release the arousal energy and get the message that it is safe to *"get up and move about the cabin."*

We may not be able to go back and redo the actual experience, nor do we need to, as this can be re-traumatizing, but God has given us a powerful way to tap into the fight-or-flight response to restore our sense of security. We have to learn how to tap back into our instinctual responses, arouse our deep physiological resources, and utilize them. *"When we harness these instincts, we can use our conscious mind to transform traumatic symptoms into a*

---

21 Levine, Peter A. *Waking the Tiger: Healing Trauma: The Innate Capacity to Transform Overwhelming Experiences.* North Atlantic Books, 1997

state of well-being."[22] The "paralysis" I experienced when I was home alone was a sign of an incomplete physiological response suspended in fear.

Reclaiming Power in Everyday Life

As I was studying this the other night, I was hit with the realization that I had been in a freeze response for several months while writing this book. My brain had been seeing this project as a threat and shutting me down to protect me. This learned habit referred to as "Overwhelm Freeze," is common when we have a huge thing to accomplish that really matters to us, and we're stumped on how to even begin. Our brain acts like it's a rabbit that's just sensed a dog in the yard and stops dead in its tracks.

I started researching this to grow in my own self-awareness and found that people who struggle with perfectionism are especially prone to it. When we over-identify with our performance, those tasks have a lot of weight on them! This got my attention because I have a tendency to over-identify with *"what I do"* as if it's a reflection of me. I've "enjoyed" this same lovely resistance regarding my business and website.

This *"freeze"* stress response occurs when we believe we can neither defeat the frightening, dangerous opponent nor run away. It doesn't feel safe to go either way, so we shut down and stay still, doing nothing. It's a reaction to a perceived threat that you can't seem to eliminate or put your finger on. Breaking free from this freeze response requires us to restore a sense of safety and empowerment within us. When I aligned with the resource of divine strength, I got my power back.

---

22 Levine, Peter A. *Waking the Tiger: Healing Trauma: The Innate Capacity to Transform Overwhelming Experiences.* North Atlantic Books, 1997

GOOD GIRL RX: Understand the Fear Paralyzing You to Unfreeze and Take Action

Fear often disguises itself as procrastination, avoidance, or shutdown, but beneath it lies a protective response—your body's way of keeping you safe from perceived risk or harm. The freeze response can leave you stuck, unsure of how to move forward, or powerless to act. But here's the truth: understanding the fear is the first step to reclaiming your power.

When you pause and ask yourself, *"What feels unsafe about this?"* you can begin to identify the hidden risks your system is sensing. From there, you can meet those fears with compassion, reconnect with your inner resources, and create a new path forward—one where you feel safe enough to take action. It's not about forcing yourself to move or shaming yourself for being stuck; it's about understanding what your body needs to feel safe again so you can gently take the next step.

Reflection Questions:

1. Can you recall a time when you felt frozen in fear, unable to move or take action? What sensations or cues of danger did you notice in your body?
2. If every behavior—including freezing—has a positive intention, what might your freeze response be trying to protect you from?
3. What fears or risks come up for you when you think about moving forward? How can you meet those fears with compassion?
4. What small, safe step can you take today to reconnect with your confidence and begin moving out of paralysis?

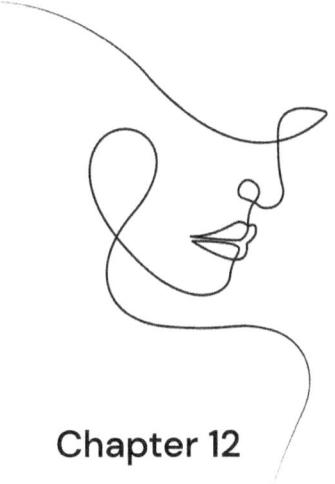

Chapter 12

From Repression to Expression: Feel to Heal

"Your repressed emotions are not trying to harm you; they're trying to tell you something. When you allow yourself to feel and express what's hidden, you make space for your body to heal."
Nicole Sachs

Jeannie's Story

When Jeannie, a sixty-year-old client, shared how she went into a three day shut down after expressing her needs and saying no to her mother it wasn't because she'd done something wrong. It was because her nervous system didn't know how to handle it. As soon as she set a boundary, shame rushed in with a vengeance.
"I'm not a good daughter,"
"I'll be judged and rejected if I assert myself,"
"I feel like I'm in a cage, and no response is okay,"
But here's the part that broke my heart. She said, "I don't tell my Christian friends about this. They'd just guilt me, give me a Sunday school answer, or say, 'pray it away.' I don't need

that. This is me breaking free. What I need is someone to ask me, *'Are you setting your boundaries? Are you standing up for yourself? You're not a bad person for doing that.'* I spent my whole life being a dutiful daughter, and I spent my whole life being rejected anyway."

At sixty, Jeannie was finally reclaiming her birthright to say no. But her body still held the story that it wasn't safe. When we find ourselves shutting down in a freeze response, the last thing we need to feel is guilt and shame. We need what was lacking when we were younger: acceptance, understanding, reassurance, and the safety to express ourselves without the fear of being judged or rejected.

Repression is the Freeze Response Continued

For many of us, the freeze response doesn't just paralyze our actions; it paralyzes our voice. What we couldn't say then becomes what we *still don't say now*, and that suppression shows up in our bodies.

All emotions are created by God for our good. Anger serves a purpose! It allows us to stand up and say "get back" when someone tries to take advantage of us. When we feel like it's not acceptable to express healthy anger, we start seething on the inside, and that suppressed anger manifests in our bodies. I did a little happy dance when I asked Jeannie what she wanted to express, and she had the courage to say, "Hell no to bottling all that up!" I think God was dancing with me.

The Hidden Cost of Emotional Repression

Suppressing emotions isn't harmless; it takes a toll on our body and mind. As Dr. John Sarno teaches, repressed emotions create tension in the body, which can manifest as chronic pain, fatigue, and illness.[23] Holding emotions in requires energy—it's like trying to hold down a pressure cooker lid as steam builds up. Eventually, it *has* to be released.

Think of it this way: Have you ever crammed things into an already overflowing cabinet? You shove and push, hoping to make it fit, but the moment you open the door—everything comes spilling out. Our bodies work the same way. Suppressed emotions don't disappear; they build up and find ways to escape. That "overflow" might look like an emotional outburst, chronic tension, migraines, or immune system suppression.

The hidden costs of emotional repression include:

- Muscle pain and tension
- Headaches and migraines
- Insomnia or restless sleep
- Digestive problems, such as stomachaches, nausea, or indigestion
- Weakened immune system, making you more susceptible to illness
- Cardiovascular issues, such as high blood pressure
- Chronic fatigue

Repression often operates beneath our awareness. It's not just the emotions we intentionally push down—that's suppression. Repression is deeper. It's what happens when we've learned so well to silence parts of ourselves that we don't even realize we're doing it. It shows up in habits like overcommitting, saying yes when we want to say no, or dismissing our own needs to avoid conflict or judgment. Over time, those unspoken "no's" and unmet needs get buried, but they don't disappear—they linger in

---

23 Dr. John Sarno explores the connection between repressed emotions and physical symptoms in *The Mindbody Prescription* and his other works. Sarno, John E. *The Mindbody Prescription: Healing the Body, Healing the Pain.* Grand Central Publishing, 1998.

our bodies, creating stress, exhaustion, and pain. That's exactly what Connie began to uncover when she shared her story.

Connie's Story

I had a client who was just beginning to make this correlation for herself without having read anything about the science of mind-body symptoms. She told me, "I don't know why I let things bother me-simple things like hosting a party. I go overboard trying to make sure everybody is happy. *So and so might not like this*, so I add something else to the menu. Then, I start stressing out about getting everything done. I don't know why I do that."

I asked, "What might be a really good reason to add more, go overboard, stress out?"

"Wanting other people to feel cared for," she replied. "I want so much for other people to be comfortable. Yet I feel no comfort. I feel pain. I've always focussed on external things to feel secure. A lady at my church passed away this week, and I was asked if I could bring a vegetable or dessert to the funeral. Instead of choosing one, I told them I could do both. If I do more, I will be accepted more. I'm taking on a lot of responsibility, and I'm tired. All my life I have tried to live up to what my mothers' expectations of me were. I've realized those expectations were wrong."

I invited her to bring compassion to the part of herself that was tired of taking on so much and speak words of life over her. Let the words she expressed that day speak life over you too-

You don't have to do all of that. You've done enough. It's okay. I'm so glad you want to help, but you need to go take a nap. Or go play for a while! Do something fun and creative that you enjoy.

Healing starts with learning to receive that comfort we're giving away to everyone else. We must take the time to pause and create space to become aware of what is happening within us. It's essential to prioritize moments for introspection, allowing us to show love and compassion to our younger selves, who may still be striving for acceptance. See that tired part of your soul as a little girl. Instead of shaming yourself for not being able to change your habits and behaviors or for getting emotional, embrace and comfort her. Those learned strategies were wired in with your early experiences–they started when you were little. That is your younger self reacting, doing more to earn acceptance and feel safe in her relationships. Your present self has a lot more wisdom and lived experience. Now you get to go back and re-parent her and give her the care she has been waiting for.

What We Resist, Persists

Emotions are energy in motion. When we suppress or repress them, they don't just go away—they linger, stored in our bodies, waiting for a release. It's like Elsa in *Frozen*: the energy erupts when we least expect it, often in destructive ways or through physical symptoms.

Here's the truth: The body doesn't forget what we suppress. As Nicole Sachs, LCSW, creator of the *JournalSpeak* method and author of *The Meaning of Truth*, says, "*The pain is not in your head, but the solution is not in your body either. The solution is in your mind.*"[24]

When we begin to honor our emotions—when we allow ourselves to feel, name, and express them—we free our bodies from the burden of holding them. Releasing what's been trapped creates space for healing.

Programmed to Repress

Many young girls learn early on that it is not safe to express themselves. When we tried to, we were reprimanded, sent away

---

24 Sachs, Nicole. *The Cure for Chronic Pain* Podcast. www.thecureforchronicpain.com.

to our rooms, shushed, or told to "suck it up." We saw people get angry or upset with us or maybe even raise a hand to us, often in the safest of homes. For others, the threat was even greater.

Maybe you learned to walk on eggshells around an abusive or emotionally fragile parent or were threatened to keep your mouth shut. Maybe you were taught to be "strong" and that crying or getting emotional was "weak," so you started covering up your vulnerability. There are countless reasons young girls become conditioned to keep it all in. We learn to self-regulate and get really good at shutting down our feelings without conscious thought. Our autonomic nervous system senses the need and activates the off switch like an underground train shifts the rail it's traveling on without the passenger's knowledge.

Self-Regulation

As a pediatric PT, I worked with children that struggled with self-regulation. Their little bodies didn't know how to contain their big feelings or impulses, and it was taking a toll on their parents, their peer relationships, and their success in school. They fidgeted, bumped into things, got overstimulated in crowded environments, screamed, and lashed out in anger when someone tried to make them do something they didn't want to.

There was one little boy who stole my heart– I still think about him from time to time and wonder how he's doing. It didn't start out that way, though. It's hard to see the heart of a child and draw near to them when their behavior makes you want to pull your hair out. Over time, I had the opportunity to develop rapport and create a sense of safety for him. I got to see the little boy behind the outbursts, hyperactivity, and disregard for directions. He was able to lower his defenses, express his true self, and regulate not only his emotion but his body.

The boy that I sat and did homework and played with was completely different from the one described by his teacher on the weekly report given to his mother. He was able to complete all the worksheets I created for him, sit at the table for fifteen minutes, follow directions, laugh, and play a game with me without getting defensive. He was smart, silly, and often really sweet.

It broke my heart to read what his teacher had written about him in the weekly report sent home to his mother. It was filled with all the things he'd done *wrong* that week: "Got up out of his seat multiple times without permission, rocked in his chair disturbing the other children, pushed someone in the hall line for standing too close to him, didn't do his work," and so much more. His mother was like, *"Don't you think I know he does these things? It doesn't help for you to record and share every 'problem' with me."* She needed some hope. She needed someone to see beyond the behaviors and hold the vision of his inherent goodness and potential.

We think the children with good behaviors and self-regulatory skills are doing great, and have report cards that say, *"Had a great day! She is wonderful to have in my class!"* Self-regulation is a really important skill for our success in society and relationships—there is no denying that—but when self regulation turns into a chronic habit of repression, the outcome is not always a good report.

Repression is the unconscious blocking of distressing thoughts, impulses, feelings, or memories out of your conscious mind, a defense mechanism designed to protect against anxiety arising from overwhelming or uncomfortable thoughts and feelings, or thoughts or emotions that are too painful to acknowledge.[25] This unconscious mechanism acts as a psychological shield to help people navigate life without the

---

25 "Repression: Psychology and Mental Health." *Verywell Health*, 13 Sept. 2023, www.verywellhealth.com/repression-7775455.

burden of distressing experiences in order to preserve emotional well-being.[26]

Suppression is a similar strategy, but happens on a conscious level, like turning away and choking back your tears. Repression, on the other hand, is entirely unconscious, making it dangerous. It's important to identify if your nervous system has developed this self-preservation strategy so you can learn to update it to one that is less health destructive.[27] If you can say yes to any of these, you might be repressing your "unacceptable" or dangerously painful emotions:

- struggling to identify and express your feelings
- emotionally distant or numb
- Unexpected mood swings, such as appearing cheerful one minute and irritable or withdrawn the next
- Avoidance of specific topics, people, or situations
- Seeking constant distractions, such as excessive work, hobbies, or screen time
- Strained relationships due to a struggle to connect emotionally, leading to communication breakdowns and misunderstandings
- Heightened stress levels
- Turning to food, alcohol, shopping, or focussing on others to try and generate feelings of comfort and escape pain
- Frequent feelings of unease, sadness, or discomfort but unable to identify the source of those feelings
- Difficulty talking about your thoughts or feelings and becoming defensive or irritated when asked about them

---

26 Oppenheimer, Steven. "Repression and the Concept of the Unconscious." *International Journal of Psychology Research*, vol. 3, no. 1, Open Access Pub, 2019, pp. 1-10, https://openaccesspub.org/ijpr/article/99.

27 "Repression: Psychology and Mental Health." *Verywell Health*, 13 Sept. 2023, www.verywellhealth.com/repression-7775455.

If the parts of our soul that are feeling scared, angry, or sad can't express themselves and an alarm goes off in our body saying, *Danger! Don't do it!* when we want to articulate our pain to others, we may give those energies no other option but to leak out and manifest in our bodies.

I love how well husband-and-wife songwriting team Kristen Anderson-Lopez and Robert Lopez expressed this in the hit song "*Let it Go*" in the movie *Frozen*.[28] There is a reason this song climbed to the top of the billboards and resonated with so many women. There is a reason why moms sat and watched it for the umpteeth time with their daughters and held out their arms in the kitchen, singing when no one was watching.

It's the message of repression and suppression that so many of us were conditioned to. We may not have had secret powers to freeze things, but our power and our voice was perceived by others to be just as threatening. Our cries, our outbursts, our opinions, our choices had the power to cause people to react and pull away. So we put on our gloves, stuffed down our authenticity, and began guarding what we expressed.

The Impact of Emotional Repression on the Body

Chronic conditions often stem from emotions we're unable to process consciously, leading our bodies to bear the burden of our unexpressed feelings. When your soul can't express itself, it will find another way to get the message through to you–often through your body.

Here are some signs your symptoms might be rooted in repression and a result of a very common mind-body neuroplastic pain syndrome, often referred to as Tension Myositis Syndrome:[29]

---

28   Lopez, Kristen Anderson, and Robert Lopez. *Let It Go*. Performed by Idina Menzel. Walt Disney Records, 2013.

29   For more information on Tension Myositis Syndrome and the mind-body connection, see:

- If you struggle with chronic pain, migraines, or other annoying symptoms and it seems like "if it's not one thing, it's another." For instance, if you have back pain for a while and then it goes away, and then it's neck pain and then that goes away, then your IBS flares up and then once *that* goes away, the cycle starts all over again.
- If the intensity fluctuates and the pain comes and goes.
- If your pain/symptoms disappear when you're busy or focused on others, but returns afterward.
- If you experience relief when you go to the beach.
- If you've tried everything to alleviate your pain and nothing is working.
- If tests keep coming back "normal" and the doctors keep telling you nothing is wrong but you are still experiencing symptoms and are obviously not okay.
- If you have had the pain/symptoms for over 6 months.
- If you've been treating the symptoms in isolation without much relief.
- If you've been blaming it on an old injury that happened more than four months ago.
- If you find yourself constantly monitoring your pain, anticipating it, or desperately asking, "*When is this ever going to go away?*"
- If you are afraid that physical activity will make your pain worse.
- If you continuously feel fearful, powerless, anxious, and/or frustrated about your symptoms.

- Sarno, John E. *Healing Back Pain: The Mind-Body Connection.* Warner Books, 1991.
- Sachs, Nicole. *The Meaning of Truth: Embrace Your Truth. Create Your Life.* Nicole J. Sachs, LCSW, 2013.
- Schubiner, Howard, and Michael Betzold. *Unlearn Your Pain.* Mind Body Publishing, 2016.

If you can answer yes to many of these signs and are ready to acknowledge the link between your chronic symptoms and the brain—embracing the mind-body connection and exploring the emotions and behavioral patterns driving them—then there is hope. Relief is possible, and there is a roadmap to guide you!

GOOD GIRL RX: Express to Heal: Release What You've Been Holding In

For many of us, embracing our emotions isn't second nature. We've learned to stay in our analytical minds and resist "feeling" as a way to stay in control and avoid what might overwhelm or consume us. This chapter is an invitation to start honoring and attending to the cries and requests of our own soul. It's about cultivating the safety for authentic expression so we can feel lighter and more carefree. Here is a fun activity to explore this.

Reflection and Creative Expression Activity:

1. Collect a few materials to draw or color with, like crayons, colored pencils, or markers—anything that feels inviting and easy to use. This doesn't need to be fancy; even a basic pencil will work.
2. Next, settle into a comfortable spot where you can focus without distractions. Take a few deep breaths, allowing yourself to slow down and tune inward.
3. Imagine that your mind and body are a foreign country you are traveling to for the first time. Bring a sense of curiosity and begin to scan around and explore it. What is it like? If it was a landscape, what would it be? A deep, dark ocean? A raging sea? A peaceful hillside? Take your pencils and have fun drawing some imagery to represent it. Don't worry about how it looks. Stick figures, basic shapes, or even just colors without any form will do.

This activity helps you develop a more compassionate connection to your body and mind. It's not about creating art but about giving shape to the inner experiences you might not have words for. The images or feelings that come up can guide you in identifying areas of tension, unprocessed emotions, or unmet needs that your body is holding onto.

Additional Resources for Deeper Exploration

Gordon, Alan, and Alon Ziv. *The Way Out: The Revolutionary, Scientifically Proven Approach to Heal Chronic Pain.* Avery Publishing, 2022.

Maté, Gabor. *When the Body Says No: The Cost of Hidden Stress.* International Version, Vermillion. 2019.

Sarno, John. *The Mindbody Prescription: Healing the Body, Healing the Pain.* Warner Books, 1998.

Sachs, Nicole. *Journal Speak Series* found on her website: https://www.yourbreakawake.com/journalspeak.

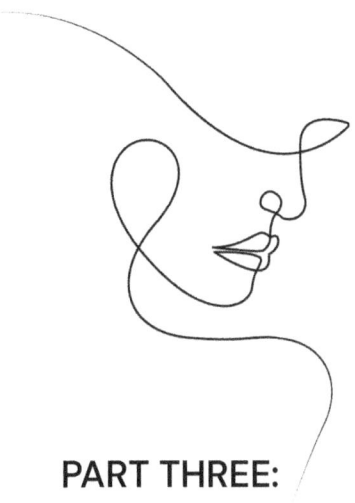

PART THREE:

THE GOOD GIRL WHO FACED HER BURIED FEARS

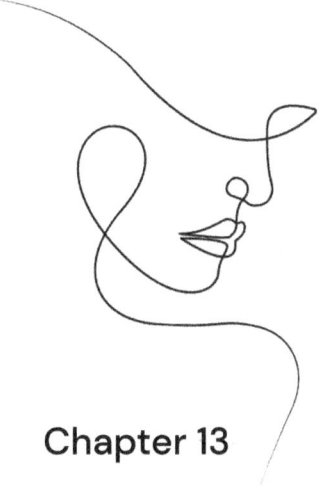

Chapter 13

Hidden Stressors: Attachment Insecurity and Codependent Patterns

"Our attachment style influences how we perceive stress, how we react to and recover from stress, and the strategies we use to cope with it."
The Attachment Project[30]

Sarah's Story: The Quest for Safety

Sarah's journey is one that resonates with so many of us—feeling anxious when we sense distance in our closest relationships. Her story speaks to the impact of attachment insecurity, where the need for constant reassurance can create hidden stressors in our minds and bodies. Through her experience, we can explore how

---

30 Summation of concepts as presented in: The Attachment Project. "Attachment Styles and Stress Responses." *The Attachment Project*, 20 June 2023, https://www.attachmentproject.com/blog/attachment-styles-and-stress-responses/.

codependent patterns arise and how learning to create safety within ourselves is key to breaking free from this cycle.

"I have this same knot in my stomach when I'm trying to communicate with my husband when I sense something's wrong," Sarah shared with me. "I can feel when he's off, especially after we've had an argument, but when I ask if he's okay, he just says, *'I'm fine.'* The more he shuts down and withdraws, the more anxious and alert I become. I start trying harder to lean in and find him; to connect. He feels that, and we feed off each other. Instead of bridging the gap, it just creates more tension. I'm getting better at not leaning in like that, but it's hard to sit in that. I need him to say, *'Sarah, you're okay. You are safe. I'm just processing. This isn't about you.'*"

Sarah continued, "If I don't know he's not upset with me, it can wreck my whole day. And if I keep getting those one word answers, and I'm not getting what I need or want from him, my wall goes up too and I just want him to go away. My anxiety and stress can get so intense, and my body feels that grip. It feels like this is my life, and I'm never going to get out of this."

"So when you're asking him if he is okay, is it about your need or his?" I asked.

"It's my need."

"How might that feel on his end?"

"Like a lot of pressure to make me feel better," she replied. "It doesn't give him the space to sit in what he's feeling."

"What if, instead of seeking reassurance from your husband, you could create that safe feeling within yourself? What if you could learn how to stay connected even when you sense him pulling back?"

"That would be great. Then my whole day wouldn't be wrecked just because someone else is feeling off."

To help Sarah break this cycle, we used a somatic exercise where I guided her to shift her attention between different sensations in her body. She started by tuning into the knot of tension in her stomach and then scanned her body until she found the steadier, more relaxed sensation in her feet resting on the floor. By going back and forth between the two—first feeling the tension in her stomach, then the grounded sensation in her feet—Sarah learned to let the grounded feeling expand, eventually filling her entire body with a sense of ease. "Wow. That feels like freedom! I have so much relief."

This exercise offered Sarah a powerful tool to manage her anxiety. She realized *I can use this when I get nervous in my stomach. It helps me shift my focus from the disconnection I'm sensing with others to my own need for peace. It also helps me feel like things can change. I don't feel trapped. I love that I can separate from their experience and come back home to myself and find me!*

Codependent Patterns and Insecurity

Sarah's deep-seated insecurities were fueling a codependent pattern where her sense of safety was tied to her husband's responses. That's not a fun place to be! Not only does our peace become hinged on the world around us, it keeps our loved ones from being able to have their own emotional experience without worrying about how it will impact us. The only way they can find separation and safety for themselves is to withdraw. Yikes! That's the opposite of what we want, isn't it?

This is a beautiful illustration of how our early attachment wounds can lead to outdated "safety" patterns that sabotage our relationships, drive internal distress, and start impacting our bodies. Sarah realized that by taking responsibility to restore her own sense of safety, she could reduce the pressure on her husband to be her emotional anchor and separate their experiences. She was able to differentiate: *This is him, and this is me. That creates safety for both of us. It doesn't put him on edge and gives him the space to deal with his own stuff, and we won't butt heads as much.*

Sarah and I discussed how this approach could help in other relationships too. She mentioned her daughter often came home from school in a bad mood. "When she slams the door, I usually let it ruin my day. But now I realize I can control my own state and not let her actions dictate my emotions."

By working on healing her early attachment insecurity, Sarah began learning how to cultivate a more stable environment for both herself and her family. It was setting the foundation to help her break free from codependent patterns that were driving her stress, her health, and relational dynamics. She shared, "This really helps me see how anxiety is driving my pain and stomach issues. When I can relieve that stress, my whole body can relax."

I understood Sarah's experience well. I have that radar that senses when others are not okay, too. It wasn't until after my oldest children had left home and I found space to heal my body that I realized just how much this had been driving my health into the ground.

My Own Journey: Sitting in the Discomfort of Feeling Disconnected

My phone vibrated, and I looked down to see my son's face pop up on the screen. I got excited... but then wondered why he was calling me. He was supposed to be on a plane headed to join his new team overseas for his first deployment. As a mom, it had been hard for me to wrap my head around his decision to join the military and defend his country, but I'd learned to make peace with it. I'd gotten a call a few years earlier when he'd hit bottom and wanted to get an appointment with a doctor to get on Adderall. "I'm a mess mom. My grades are a mess. My body is a mess. My eating habits are a mess. Even my room is a mess. I need help."

When your son, the toughest guy you know, cries out vulnerably like that, you know they're in a bad place.

He'd told us his senior year that he wanted to enlist in the military, but we convinced him to go to college first and wait until he was a little older before making that decision. It felt like such a big one. So he put it aside, got a partial scholarship to play football at a university eight hours away, and gave it his all. Nine months after that phone call and a heartbreaking season of injuries, we sat in the living room with him, trying to help him choose classes to sign up for at the community college. My husband was starting to get frustrated, as every option was met with resistance and excuses like, *"I won't be able to work enough hours if I take that class."*

I finally pressed the pause button and said, "It doesn't sound like you want to take classes. You're finding every reason not to. Is there something else you'd rather be doing?" Long pause.

"I want to join the military."

That was the moment I stopped worrying about his future and well-being. I realized I would rather see him follow his heart and pursue what he loves than live a long, miserable life trying to make others comfortable. Two months later, we gave him a hug, and he took off on a bus to basic training. It didn't surprise me when he started scoring at the top on every test, mental and physical, that he took. He used to try to tell me he just wasn't as smart as his sister, who was her class valedictorian, but I knew different. I knew it had nothing to do with his ability and everything to do with his motivation. The reason he started excelling and was able to lead his class in the Soldier's Creed at their graduation was because he cared about what he was doing. It mattered to him. He had chosen this.

Fast forward to the day my phone rang. I answered and heard on the other end, "They canceled my flight. They're sending me back home. I'm landing in Nashville this afternoon. Can someone come get me?"

"Of course. I'll be there. I'm so sorry."

Part of me was relieved, but another part grieved for him. I knew he'd felt lost the last month waiting around to be connected to a team with no sense of purpose or belonging. I couldn't imagine what this setback felt like for him, but I knew having to call your mom to come get you when you were just about to step into your purpose wasn't on his bucket list.

I was sitting at a coffee shop near his gate, watching for him, when my heart leaped as I saw him approaching in his uniform. I stood up from my stool to greet him, wanting to wrap my arms around him, but instead, he glanced my way and kept walking. I saw that another guy from his team that was in the same situation was walking alongside him and thought, he's just embarrassed. Respect his need for space. I followed him through the airport, each of us pulling along our own stuff. He dragged his duffle bag while I kept my emotions zipped up, feeling like I was tucking my heart into my own carry-on.

As I drove down the highway toward our home, my brain searched for something I could say to ease the tension, interrupt the silence, and lower the wall between us. I'd learned a lot about myself at this point and knew I needed to give him space to feel what he was feeling. I knew what I was experiencing in my body was more about my own discomfort. His distance had nothing to do with me, but that didn't make it any easier. My body still registered it as rejection. It felt like he did not want to be riding in that truck with me.

I'd spent my whole life working to bridge those gaps and make people feel more at ease so I could connect with them, so sitting there trying to will myself to keep my mouth shut was like trying to walk across a bed of nails. I reached my pain tolerance after an hour of fighting that internal battle and finally shouted, "I know this sucks, and I can't imagine what this must be like for you, but say something, anything! Scream if you want to! I can't stand this!" I can't remember exactly what he said that day, but I caught the most important thing:

"Mom, this isn't about you!"

I needed to hear that again. It was my cue to realize I still had more of my own work to do. He stayed with us several days before he got instructions for his next steps, and I used it as an opportunity to do things differently.

One morning, I saw him sitting at the table. My first impulse was to join him and engage in conversation, but I paused. Even though that felt like the "right" thing to do, I pivoted. I took my yogurt and coffee to the dining room and leaned into some work. I wasn't getting much work done because everything in me was wrestling with that decision, feeling like I was not a good mom—that I should be spending what little time I had with my son, showing interest in him. But I breathed through it and stayed where I was, letting it be okay for us to be in separate rooms. After about an hour, he approached me and started having a conversation.

That was a huge lightbulb moment for me and a corrective experience that served to show me what happens when we ground ourselves in love instead of moving toward people in anxiety. By sitting in the tension of my compulsive need to lean in, I cultivated a safer environment for him to have his own experience and come to me in his own time.

I realized when I was working on fine-tuning the messaging for this book that this was the most important work I have done. This is the thing that has had the most radical influence on my own well-being and has served to change the relational dynamics between me and my children. I'm still a work in progress, but the fact that I can be at peace and feel nothing but happiness for my children that are serving overseas and living miles away from me is a testament to what can happen when we do the work to heal our own insecurities.

As much as I love the freedom and peace that comes with that on my end, it's the freedom I pray my kids feel that means the most to me. I want my daughter to be able to call me and celebrate my granddaughter's new words and be able to tell me about things they are doing without feeling sad or like I'm missing out. I know what that feels like to be on the receiving end of that. You stop sharing because you know you'll just be met with, *"I wish I could be there."* It becomes about my own unmet needs and sabotages the experience she was trying to reach out and share.

I know that as my son got older, he learned to guard his emotions so I wouldn't be impacted by them. It breaks my heart to know that his patterns of avoidance likely developed from his own need for safety–that it didn't feel safe for him to feel what he was feeling around me. Every time he got anxious, angry, or upset, I swooped in to try and alleviate it, but just like Sarah, instead of restoring peace, it often escalated everything. When our kids or loved ones withdraw, they aren't doing it to hurt us. They may be shutting us out to create the separation they need for their own well-being and because they know expressing it will just upset us. I don't think it's what they want any more than taking on responsibility for everyone else's emotions is what we want. Whether it's anxiety or avoidance, both patterns sabotage what we're going for: the safety to be ourselves in a room and feel deeply connected.

We want so badly for them to lower their wall and let us in, but until we start understanding how that feels on their end, we will continue to endure the heartbreak of distance and one-sided relationships. Our need for them to lower the wall is our *own* need. My son was right. What was going on for him was not about me but what was going on *within* me. The solution is to stop trying so hard to lower their wall or bridge that gap and shift our attention to ourselves.

I don't know about you, but I was taught that that was selfish. Can you see the opposite is true? What I did in the car that day was all about me. I may have cared about what he was going through and wished I could take it away, but my need to invade his privacy superseded his need to ride quietly in the truck next to someone who wasn't threatened by the silence. Moving toward people out of a compulsive need to fix what we are feeling is rooted in fear and insecurity—and they can sense that. We think we're leaning in to love them, but we're not.

If this resonates with you, I'm sending you a lot of compassion and a big hug. This is a hard pill to swallow, but one too important to bypass. I know how much your relationships mean to you, and as heartbreaking as it is to awaken to this awareness, it's also a beautiful opportunity. Nothing changes without the awareness of what is happening unconsciously.

I used to think that the tension and conflict in my life came from "the enemy" or outside forces working against me. What I came to realize is that the enemy I'd been blaming wasn't some supernatural force but a scared little girl inside me whose ego was trying to protect her.

When we learn to associate helping with being loved, helping feels like the right thing to do. However, when we shift from seeking love through helping to offering help from a place of security, we move from insecurity to genuine connection, setting the stage for deeper and more authentic relationships. Fear pushes people away; love draws them in. When we start loving our fearful parts and attending to them as Sarah did that day, our protectors can relax their grip on our lives, giving us space to heal and step into spirit-led self-leadership.

GOOD GIRL RX: Heal Your Attachment Wounds

When we heal our attachment wounds, we can discover a love so profound that it holds our fears and insecurities with compassion. This love isn't something we merely seek outside ourselves but a presence we embody, becoming not only anchors of safety but conduits of that love. In learning to extend this love to ourselves, we become ambassadors of peace within, opening a pathway to unshakable calm in our hearts, relationships, and lives.

Reflection Questions:

1. Reflect on the patterns of attachment insecurity and codependency that Sarah experienced. Do you recognize any similar tendencies in yourself? How does your need for reassurance from others show up in your relationships?
2. How do your own attachment patterns impact your physical health, stress, or emotional well-being? Do you notice tension, anxiety, or digestive issues like Sarah did? What is your body trying to tell you about the hidden stressors you're carrying?
3. Take a moment to reflect on your relationships. Is there anywhere you've placed the responsibility for your emotional safety onto someone else? How might it feel to create a safe, grounded space within yourself instead of needing to rely on external validation or reassurance?

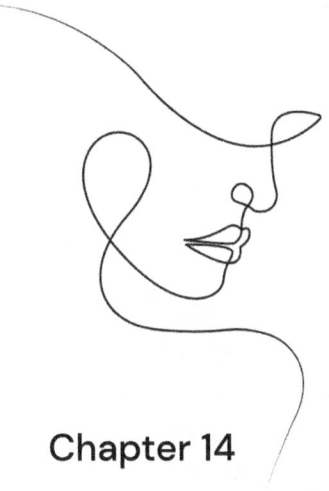

Chapter 14

Unraveling Anxiety: Hypervigilance and Restoring a Sense of Security

"Anxiety isn't just in your mind. It's your body trying to protect you from past pain projected into the future."
Dr. Russell Kennedy[31]

Much like Sarah, I had my own battles with anxiety that often surfaced in physical ways. One night, I got really lightheaded and clammy with sharp pains in my stomach that took me to my knees. When I felt stable enough, I climbed the stairs to my bedroom, carrying my silent fears with me. My husband asked if I needed to go to the ER, but I had no desire to repeat my previous experience and be treated like the boy crying

---

31   Kennedy, Dr. Russell, host. *The Anxiety Rx Podcast.* 2021, Spotify, https://open.spotify.com/show/4IYqkiwRF5GGoolW6F2odj.

wolf, so I curled up and cried, praying to God that the pain would calm and nothing was seriously wrong.

I made an appointment with my gynecologist the next day to at least go in and find out why I'd been having so much pain. They scheduled an ultrasound the following week that showed I had ovarian cysts and had likely experienced one rupturing the night I collapsed in pain. The nurse said the cysts were "complex" and gave me the option of following up in three months, giving them a chance to resolve, or removing my ovaries if I was done having children. I went home and googled "complex cysts" to better understand what I was dealing with. I didn't like what I found. Apparently, complex cysts are the kind that often become cancerous. That's not something you want to read when your subconscious remembers that taking radioactive iodine for thyroid cancer came with an increased risk for a secondary cancer to develop.

I shared my fears with my doctor, and she scheduled a CA 125 blood test that detects protein levels often found in women with ovarian cancer. When I got the call telling me the levels were slightly elevated, there was no question in my mind that I wanted to schedule the surgery ASAP. I didn't get a second opinion or even consider if the results might be due to something less threatening like endometriosis. I had no desire to give it a few months and see if the cysts would dissolve naturally. My brain wasn't looking for other possibilities. All it heard was *"cancer risk,"* and it was shouting, *get them out of our body now!*

They put me on birth control pills in the meantime, as that was standard treatment for ovarian cysts, but all that did was freak me out more. I started having new scary symptoms, like extreme bloating and "bumps" on my breast. All the things I'd read about as potential signs of ovarian cancer were found by my brain, confirming the evidence it was watching and scanning for. I couldn't get that surgery fast enough.

I awoke after the procedure to learn that I didn't have cancer or complex cysts after all. In fact, one ovary had been fine and the other just had some endometriosis around it. The cysts they had seen in the ultrasound had, in fact, resolved. People told me I should have been thanking God and seeing this as an answered prayer, but it didn't feel that way to me.

I knew that fear had driven me to remove parts from my body as if they were an enemy attacking me and threatening my life. I knew that I'd allowed my past to be projected onto my future, and I'd rushed into doing something without looking for other possibilities. I was so laser focused on what might be wrong that I didn't stop to consider or even look for what might be naturally occurring and explore more conservative options. I let my actions be hijacked by my fear centers, and I woke up mad at the world for it. I was angry at my doctor for not leaving my one good ovary, and I was upset about going into early menopause unnecessarily. It was the same fear that used to send me running back up the basement stairs if I heard a sound and couldn't see who made it–the same fear that left me feeling lonely when no one was around to reassure me.

We don't like the unknown. It feels dangerous, and our nervous systems go on high alert to protect us. When we've had scary health experiences, it's easy to become hypervigilant and attuned to signs of danger. The problem is this vigilance can backfire. We start chasing symptoms and seeing our bodies as threatening when what we need most is to restore our sense of safety.

As long as we continue to run away from or fight our symptoms—trying to suppress or eliminate them—we will remain stuck in survival mode. This sends danger signals to our brains and bodies, making them believe we are in crisis. Our nervous systems receive this message, and all systems turn off to respond to the life threat. *She doesn't need to reproduce, digest, or sleep right now. Her life is in danger! Eliminate all contents from her bladder and bowels so she can run faster without being distracted by that!* Can you see why it might make sense to have bloating, urinary urgency, or loose bowels in that context?

Our thoughts are powerful. Our minds and bodies are always communicating like faithful pen pals, sharing all their secrets and responding as quickly as they can.

Sarah's Story: Connecting Health and Stress

Sarah's relationship with her health had been complex, fraught with the same anxiety I experienced. However, Sarah's anxiety had been a life-long battle. She'd experienced a large range of symptoms and spent a considerable amount of time and energy trying to understand and resolve them, keeping her in a cycle of worry and insecurity. In one of her first sessions with me, I led her in a body scan to help her connect more deeply with her internal world so she could gain clarity on the root of her symptoms. As I invited her to let go and allow herself to be held by the chair and settle into the present moment, she admitted how hard that was for her: "I don't do that. I keep going, doing—always under pressure."

I encouraged her to breathe deeply and simply notice her sensations without trying to fix or change anything. As she began to relax, she reported: "There's tension and discomfort, but as I keep breathing and just noticing, it starts to release on its own."

Sarah's left shoulder, which had been particularly tense despite regular massages, began to soften. She reflected, "When I was at my parent's house last week, my body was tensing up, and I realized I was constipated. I've had stomach issues ever since I was a kid and even had to get a colonoscopy. This is the first time I'm connecting it to stress, not just the food I ate." This realization was profound for her. She began to see how her childhood stress responses were still affecting her adult body: "My younger self is able to understand her body now. I can give myself grace instead of getting mad at myself."

The Care We Expect to Receive

Sarah recognized that she was adding more to her plate with all the appointments, escalating her stress rather than addressing the root causes. She shared how she recently had a bump that came and went at her hernia site and how she'd asked her husband to look at it to make sure she was okay. She went on to share that her father would often catastrophize health issues: "He'd say a headache might be cancer, so I'd always think I had to get everything checked out." Sarah realized that this hypervigilance was exhausting: "If that part of me didn't have to be so watchful and alert, I could breathe..."

As an action step, she decided to show appreciation to her protective part and wrote a letter to her body. She acknowledged how much time she spent under the medical microscope—heart ablation, nose surgeries, hernia repairs, skin issues—and expressed her fatigue with this cycle: "I'm done. I'm over this." She also realized a deeper need underneath her health anxiety and hypervigilance. "I need to feel heard and like I matter. If something happens medically and I miss it, I need to know someone cares."

I see this subconscious association in many of my clients. Our relationship to our primary caregivers and the way they attended to us when we were sick as children plays a large role in our current relationship with our bodies and what we're feeling in them. Sarah's experience is a prime example of this. If our parents respond to our falls, our bumps, our moles, or are fevers with anxiousness and urgency, our bodies become wired to expect that kind of attention when we're sick or hurting as adults, even if it feels like too much.

My own mother may have been busy and not always available, but when I was sick, she was right there doting on me, calling the doctor and forcing me to drink Alka Seltzer. She even took me to the doctor to investigate a bump on my chest that turned out to be my breast bud developing; talk about humiliating. As much as I hated her hovering, it was familiar for me. As an adult, I struggled with the absence of that attention. My husband didn't have that same awareness and never even noticed when I was crying. It was like going from one extreme to the other. I felt more secure with him because he didn't need or hover over me, but my nervous system also saw his lack of engagement as threatening. I'd come to expect more care and attention when I was sick, even if it was suffocating.

I think this is the reason I had so much insecurity arise anytime I was sick, hurting, or feeling vulnerable. I handled everything myself, but I'd find myself crying, *Mommy, I need you,* from my bathroom floor when I was in agony with cramps or after throwing up all night. I wanted to maintain my independence and not depend on anyone, but when I did, I felt alone and uncared for. There was a push and pull dynamic: *I don't need you. Yes I do. I want you, but it doesn't feel safe to need you.*

These attachment dynamics around our health experiences play a huge and often overlooked role in our outcomes. If we can't feel safe, our nervous system can't regulate, and we can't relax into rest and repair. If we see every symptom as a threat or are unable to rest or reach out for support when we're sick, we will stay dysregulated and get caught in a cycle of distress and overwhelm. Our health will take a hit. The most important ingredient to our relationships and healing is restoring an internal sense of security. Fear and anxiety may be helpful when there is an emergency, but chronic patterns steal, kill, and destroy everything in their path.

Sarah discovered that her protective energy could be redirected toward more positive activities—having fun, being creative, enjoying herself, feeling free, dancing, and listening to music. "Using that energy for joy would reduce my stress, lower my blood pressure, and help my body stay safe without feeling so heavy." This shift in perspective allowed Sarah to see that creating a sense of safety within herself, rather than constantly seeking reassurance from medical appointments, could lead to a more balanced and fulfilling life. I learned this, too. It wasn't until I stopped funneling all my energy and attention into trying to fix my body and shifted my focus on my soul that my body started settling. One day I just went, *Huh. Isn't that interesting. I'm not hurting anymore.*

Codependency and Our Bodies: The Vicious Cycle

During one session, Sarah shared that she noticed some new bumps arising around an incision site and then started having a lot of bloating, amplifying her fear that something wasn't right in her body. She'd gone on a liquid diet as her stomach was responding sensitively to everything she tried to eat. "All it takes is five chips, and I bloat. It's not the amount of food or even a type of food."

"When did you first notice that?" I asked.

"About a month ago."

"Was it before you noticed the bumps or after?"

"After," Sarah replied.

"Hmm, let's approach this with curiosity," I suggested. "I wonder what let your body know to start bloating after you discovered those bumps? What might have let the body know you were under threat and that digesting food might not be a good idea right now?"

She started realizing her relationship to her body was very similar to her relationship to others when they were suffering. She saw a problem and wanted to fix it, solve it, and make it go away. There was a sense of urgency and anxiety that was amplifying her fears and symptoms instead of bringing the calm reassurance she needed to feel safe. The more she shared her health fears with others that had this same urgency, the more her fear was fed.

How we do one thing is how we do everything. The way we relate to others becomes the way we relate to our bodies. If we can't tolerate the suffering of others without feeling the need to fix it for them, we may not be able to tolerate our own suffering without going into the same anxious attachment pattern of trying to fix ourselves to escape the unease.

The anxiety that fuels codependency in relationships can also fuel a fixation on our symptoms. If we see them as problems to be solved rather than signals to be understood, we can get caught in a relentless cycle of self-improvement that becomes more harmful than helpful. This drive to "fix" ourselves to alleviate anxiety makes us hyper-focused on our symptoms, driven by the same urgency to "fix" ourselves that we apply to fixing others. Codependency locks us into a survival pattern where we are constantly reacting to perceived threats, whether they come from others or from within our own bodies. This can lead to excessive treatments, medications, and hypervigilance that often exacerbate the very symptoms we're trying to alleviate.

GOOD GIRL RX: Break Free From the Fixation Trap

When we shift our focus from what needs "solved" to what nourishes and fulfills us, we break free from survival mode into a state of peace and restoration. Take a moment to reflect on the questions below and consider how codependent patterns might be contributing to your distress and how you can start untangling from it.

Reflection Questions:

1. What areas of your life do you find yourself constantly trying to fix, solve, or control? Write down any specific symptoms, situations, or relationships where you tend to focus your energy on finding solutions or preventing problems. How does this impact your sense of peace and presence?
2. Where does codependency show up in your life, especially when it comes to the need to fix others or seek reassurance? Reflect on any relationships where you tend to prioritize the needs of others or their emotions over your own. How might this drive your need for control or contribute to anxiety?
3. What is one small action you could take this week to redirect your attention toward something that brings you joy or peace? Make a commitment to notice when you go into "fixing" mode and gently guide your focus to something that nourishes and restores your energy. What might that look like for you?

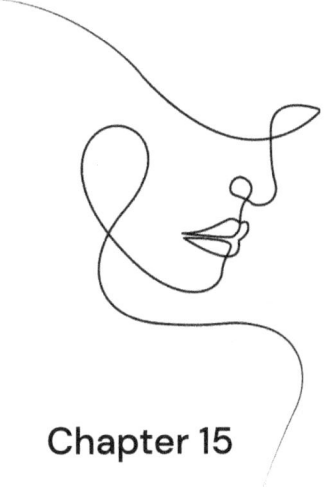

Chapter 15

Finding Freedom in Setting Boundaries

"Boundaries are the distance at which I can love you and me simultaneously."
Prentis Hemphill[32]

Have you ever been told by a doctor or well-meaning friend, *"You just need to start setting boundaries. Say 'no' more. Stop committing to so much. You really should take better care of yourself. You need to reduce your stress."* If only it was that easy, right?

It's not a matter of just being more intentional. It's not even about time management. You can identify your priorities, time block your calendar, and ask God for strength all day long, but as soon as you sense someone is "not okay," upset with you, or are informed of a need, you're like a child being dragged away from the playground against their will with no power to resist the pull. A part of you longs to open up time to breathe, rest, and pursue

---

32   Commonly attributed but not verified.

your passions, but another part hijacks your plan and moves into action to take on responsibility–again.

Women often get mad at God, blaming others or the enemy when some new need, situation, crisis, or expectation gets in the way of their desires. It can be very disheartening when things don't work out, making you feel like it's just not meant to be. We often find ourselves thinking, *I guess that just wasn't God's will for me. I must have misunderstood His intentions. Surely, if it was meant to be, He would open a door, create a way for me, and grant me peace.* The truth is, it often feels unsafe to pursue what we truly desire. You might find yourself feeling excited and optimistic after taking a step back or agreeing to something new. Everything seems to be going well, but then suddenly, a setback occurs—like your car breaking down, a coworker falling ill, or your husband or child becoming distant. In these moments, your inner "protector" kicks in, sounding the alarm. You start to feel that someone else is not okay, and your instinct tells you to abort your plans and go fix the situation. We self-abandon to restore peace.

Why does this happen? Remember the little girl who learned to connect with others by paying attention to her surroundings? She learned how to respond in ways that made the room feel less stressful. That same survival strategy is the reason setting boundaries can be so difficult. If we don't respond, that same vulnerability and fear of abandonment starts churning in our chest. If we don't fix it, we will continue to feel the insecurity and disconnection that we experienced as children. The strategies we learn to survive become the strategies upon which our continued survival depends upon. Your brain knows this strategy has worked so far, but it doesn't know what might happen if you try something new. When you feel something dangerous and risky, a part of your amygdala—the part of your brain responsible for evaluating danger—alerts you, signaling that you need to take action to escape that feeling. That energy you start feeling–that urgency–that's not God, and it's not the enemy. It's your fear centers, doing what they are designed to do: protect your vulnerability. Your survival brain thinks it's helping you, but its methods are often outdated, comparing the incoming information with all your old memories and the emotions stored with them. Instead of keeping you alive, it's often tanking your energy and derailing you from your dreams. The good news is that there is a way to break free from this unconscious self-sabotage and start setting boundaries with confidence and strength. You have the power to reclaim your energy and realign with your dreams.

Our Inner Protectors

I love when my clients introduce me to their "protective parts." They call them names like Steve and describe them as big, burly guys, bouncers, or defendant attorneys. It's the masculine energy that holds their power and confidence. They're like big brothers, overprotective fathers, and brave soldiers standing guard, using all their energy and attention to safeguard you. The problem is that they often won't let you do anything. You're stuck in your room while they respond to every little threat, telling you, *"Sorry, but it's just not safe for you to go to that party or pursue that dream."* Or worse, they keep telling you you have to clean the house better, sign up for the PTA, volunteer for the church nursery, make a homemade meal, call your mother every day, go back to that job that sucked the life out of you so your family doesn't feel any strain, and skip the walk on the beach you wanted to take because you should be spending more time with your kids.

Protective energy is not the same thing as personal power and confidence. The first flows from fear, the latter from love and security. When we are aligned with love, we can stand in our power and assert ourselves without having to get in someone's face and demand to be heard. Learning to say no and setting powerful boundaries around your time, energy, and attention doesn't mean you have to go over to the "dark side" and become mean, invasive, or bossy. True power always produces fruit. Power rooted in fear destroys relationships.

Managers and Firefighters

I love how Richard Schwartz, founder of the Internal Family Systems Theory, explains the protective parts of our soul, dividing them into two types: Managers and Firefighters.[33] They both have similar motivations, but one works on the front end to prevent "the fire" and the other when it's already underway. The "Good Girl" is managing things through her people-pleasing, kindness, caring, and appropriate behaviors, but if a fire erupts anyway, the "Bad Girl" comes out with her hose. You know your manager is on the scene when you are tippy-toeing around someone, holding back your words, shrinking away from conflict, overcommitting your time and energy, deflecting compliments, over apologizing, pushing yourself to do more when your body is clearly in need of some downtime, or saying yes to making your daughter's favorite meal when she begs you even though you had a really rough week and would really prefer to order take out. Your firefighter has come racing in on the truck when you're slamming doors, hanging up on your mom, going back into the room for the third time to make sure your point is heard, grabbing the ice cream and a spoon to drown your emotions, and then forcing yourself to go to the gym as punishment afterward.

The thing to remember is that these lovely protectors are just trying to keep you alive. They are important parts of you and deserve appreciation for all they have done. You might not be here today if they hadn't learned those strategies. At one point, they were necessary. When we get to know and befriend these

---

33 Schwartz, Richard C. *Internal Family Systems Therapy*. Guilford Press, 1995. See also Schwartz, Richard C. *No Bad Parts: Healing Trauma and Restoring Wholeness with the Internal Family Systems Model*. Sounds True, 2021.

parts, they become more supportive and less self-sabotaging. Your inner critic can become your cheerleader, and your door slammer becomes your advocate, communicating with assertion on the front end instead of fixing problems later.

My self-doubting part, when I remind it, now uses its energy to help me trust myself, stop overthinking, and make confident decisions. In the same way we tell our children that their bossiness can turn into a beautiful gift of leadership, our protectors can learn to use their energy for good in the world.

Just like campaign teams work tirelessly behind the scenes to secure a candidate's victory, our internal managers and firefighters coordinate efforts to protect and preserve our well-being. When we understand their motives, align their efforts with our true needs, and harness their energy positively, they become like trusted campaign aides, channeling their dedication into constructive action and orchestrating a winning strategy for our well-being.

Challenging Our Fears Around Setting Boundaries

When I first started trying to set boundaries around my time as a business owner, I was worried I'd be seen as rude or uncaring. I was so used to giving my undivided attention and personal touch that delegating communication to someone else felt scary. My coach encouraged me to try a marketing and outreach company she was using. This would allow me to focus on serving my current clients and creating resources for them rather than spending so much time communicating with women who weren't seeking support or ready to invest. I decided to give it a try. I worked with them to craft the messaging I wanted to share, along with an offer for a free strategy session.

The company warned me to step back once it got in motion and let the team do their job—in other words, not to micromanage them—but man, was that hard! I couldn't help peeking at the way the message was being received. One day, I noticed a woman sharing her struggles with a recent cancer diagnosis, and when I saw the response to her, I freaked out. Yikes! They weren't showing as much empathy as I would have, and it wasn't sitting well with me. I immediately shared my concern about how I'd prefer they respond in the future. It wasn't that there was anything wrong with teaching them to communicate with the women in a way that best represented my business. I did need to do that. But I also needed to give them space to learn and let go of a few things without feeling like the world was going to come crashing down if someone got offended.

On my coaching call the next day, my coach asked me, "What is the fear?"

"That they will think I'm rude and uncaring."

"If you really care about serving the women that invest in your services at the highest level and guarding your energy for them, you're going to have to learn to get unhinged from what everyone else thinks about you."

Truth bomb. I sat and received it.

She was right. If I spent all my time responding and worrying about people God hadn't even called or equipped me to serve, I was going to stay scattered and frustrated. I was spending so much energy speaking and communicating with people who weren't even looking for my help. I'd catch myself going down rabbit holes in Facebook groups responding to people's questions and realize I'd just wasted an hour of my day that I'd intended for something else. My protective, empathetic part just couldn't help herself. If she saw someone in need, she felt compelled to respond. She meant well, but she was sabotaging my "yes" and the work I felt called to. We do not have the bandwidth to respond to everyone.

We have to get unhinged from our insecurity and fear of rejection, or we'll continue to feel scattered, frustrated, and resentful. When we expand our capacity to feel discomfort by sitting with ourselves in compassion, we find the acceptance and reassurance we needed all along. If you're feeling scattered, drained, or over-committed, those are red flags that it's time to pivot your attention. It's time to listen and respond to your own soul.

Getting Clear on Our Yes

Boundaries are like guardrails on the highway that guide us toward our destination. We often struggle to set these boundaries because we aren't clear about what we are protecting. We need to recognize that our "yes" is so important that we must be willing to say "no" to everything else that could interfere with it. When we know the reason for our "yes," the "no's" get easier. We no longer see boundaries as rude but necessary for protecting what we value most. When we overextend ourselves, trying to please everyone, we end up not serving anyone well, often hurting those we love the most. I could keep doing what I was doing, but unless I learned to let it go, I would never attract ideal clients, be fairly paid for my services, and do the work my soul felt drawn to.

I'll never forget the first time I got a notification on my phone that someone had signed up for a session without me lifting a finger. I was away on vacation with my family and thought, *Wow, that's crazy! My business is working for me while I'm gone. The decision to invest in delegating and put boundaries around my empathy was paying off!*

When I got back, I had three sessions booked, and at the end of the call, all three eagerly said "yes" to investing in the results they wanted. Not only did that lead me to a month of my highest profits, but the opportunity to support some amazing women and witness them stepping into results that were their highest priority.

If I hadn't learned to sit in the discomfort I felt in setting those boundaries and overcoming my fear, I would probably still be working as a PT right now and never have written this book. It's not that I couldn't help people in that context, but I realized that what God had been teaching me through my experiences, training, and research was far too important to let my fears hold me back. I couldn't help other women embrace their own paths if I didn't first learn to set boundaries for myself.

Internal Boundaries

There are a lot of great books out there on how to set boundaries, but what I've discovered personally and professionally is that trying to set boundaries with others before learning how to set boundaries with ourselves is like putting the cart before the horse: we don't get anywhere. As long as shame, guilt, insecurity, and our fierce inner critics are running the show, trying to set boundaries around your time and energy is like trying to walk with your shoelaces tied together. You're going to trip every time and come away with bruises.

We need to learn how to engage with the different parts of our soul so that they can step back and allow us the space we need. By establishing and respecting our boundaries, these parts can stop sabotaging us. When we embrace self-leadership and become the fantastic bosses of our own lives—recognizing our potential—these aspects of ourselves become eager to support us. Instead of creating internal conflicts, they begin to work together toward peace, freedom, and empowered action in the world. This is the support you've been longing for, even if you didn't realize you had access to it. Best of all, they don't require any payment—just your appreciation and respect.

Dr. Allusion Cook, PhD and Author of Boundaries Around Your Soul translates this model of the soul through a Christian lens, showing us how to love our internal enemies in the same way Jesus taught us to love those that persecute us: "But I tell you, love your enemies and pray for those who persecute you"

(Matthew 5:44). It's a wonderful read, and the insights and understanding she brings have been game changers in my own life.

When we learn to lead, care for, and understand our own souls, we become strong inside. We are able to respond to life's challenges with greater resilience and become true to the person God created us to be and the work he planned for us to do. Dr Cook shares the recipe for powerful boundaries, stating, "You'll be realistic about your limitations and have a clear sense of your own values, vision, mission and priorities. You'll understand the health of your relationships and the sustainability of your service depends on your ability to make wise decisions about how you spend your time."[34] This is what spiritual formation is all about! Powerful boundaries are always the byproduct of self-leadership and care.

GOOD GIRL RX: Honor Your Yes With Powerful Boundaries

Setting boundaries can be challenging, especially when old patterns and protective parts step in. As you reflect on this chapter, take a moment to identify what's been getting in the way of setting boundaries so you can create the space to honor your "yes" and align your life with what truly matters.

---

34 Cook, Alison, and Kimberly Miller. *Boundaries for Your Soul: How to Turn Your Overwhelming Thoughts and Feelings into Your Greatest Allies*. Thomas Nelson, 2018.

Reflection Questions:

1. Can you identify a recent time when you overcommitted or self-abandoned in response to someone else's needs? How did this affect your energy, well-being, or plans? What were the beliefs, feelings, or fears underneath your response?
2. Are there areas of your life where you're giving your energy to things or people that aren't aligned with your true purpose? How might setting boundaries in those areas free up energy for your most important "yes"?
3. Take a moment to reflect on what truly matters to you. What is the "yes" your body and soul are inviting you to prioritize in this season? How can setting boundaries protect and honor that?

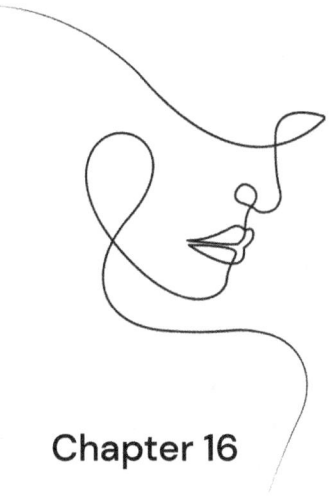

Chapter 16

Breaking Free From Self Sabotage

"Believe you can and you're halfway there."
Theodore Roosevelt

My daughter's body sat a little taller as her confidence returned and hope filled her back up again. Moments before, she'd ripped off her sweatshirt after spilling water on it and declared, "I can't go to school. I feel awful. I'm hot and itchy and my stomach hurts. I'm tired and I didn't sleep well." Then she dropped herself in the chair, leaning her head on her hands in defeat. My heart went out to her, but there was also a part of me going, "Not again. She needs to go to school." I paused to align myself and check in to see what love would do. My first thought was, "Give her some time. Let her be. She's already found a way to calm herself. Just give her a minute." After some time had passed, I walked up, hugged her gently, and whispered, "I'm sorry you're feeling bad. You had a rough night last night, yeah?"

"It was fine. I'm used to it," she replied from the hole in the pretzel her arms were creating around her. We discussed her need to go to school and how she feels this way frequently when she is upset but usually feels better later. That was me trying to help her connect the dots between what she was feeling physically and what was brewing under the surface, not being given a voice. Maybe not the best strategy, but I was trying, looking for what landed and what didn't. She'd gone to a dance audition the night before and was the only one in her level, along with some younger dancers, to not get a call back. She'd come home and shared the news matter of factly, but never showed any emotion around it as she had in previous experiences like this. I could tell she was numbing herself and going into that "It is what it is" mode that we often adopt when we're trying to accept something. But in actuality, she was shutting down her desire to get away from the pain of defeat. I paused again, then replied, "Hmm, if I had had that happen to me, that would have stung." She replied, "Well, yeah, but I'm used to it by now. They're never going to choose me. I don't have the flexibility like the other girls, and I'm never going to be as good as them."

"Hmm," I paused again, letting that sit in the room, then asked gently, "Would you say that to a friend?"

"Well, no."

"Did you want to make it? Do you want to excel at dance?"

"Well, that's why I did the audition. I did want it," she admitted. "I know that if I was just given a chance, I could learn the choreography and do really well."

"Yeah, I believe that too. Can I ask you a question?" I looked up to check for confirmation, then proceeded: "It feels like there's a part of you that loves dance and wants to excel at it, and another part that's telling you you're not good enough and that part isn't letting you work for something you want? Does that feel true?"

"Yeah, I do love dancing." Long pause..."I was looking at old videos from when I was younger, and I was on the front row a lot."

"Yeah you were," I agreed. "You used to believe in yourself. What shifted?"

"The teachers started putting me in the back, and I started feeling like I wasn't as good."

"It sounds like you lost faith in yourself," I replied. "Do you think a part of you might hold you back from pursuing what you want because it still believes that no matter how hard you try, you'll never be good enough?"

She sat with that. No reply needed.

"Baby, those teachers that used to put you in the front row still believe in you, but it doesn't matter how much they or I encourage you if you don't believe in yourself. It's up to you to choose to support yourself and give yourself the chance to excel if this is something you really want."

"But, it's too late. I can't catch up."

"It's never too late," I encouraged. "You have two more years, and even if you never make an audition piece, you still have the opportunity to work toward your full potential. Remind me what you love about dance? Is it something you want to continue, or is there something else you'd rather be working toward?"

"Well, I'd love to be on the dance team in college, and I just found out Auburn has a show choir. I really love choir, and I do want to try theater next year," she replied.

"Consider what you might need to let go of to pursue what you truly want to do. Are you dancing because it's something you've always done, and you feel you can't stop because you said you wouldn't?"

"I told myself I'd never quit!" she exclaimed.

"Then don't quit. But what if, instead of being so loyal to dance, you started being loyal to yourself? Give yourself permission to support yourself fully and work for the things that make you happy." As we both sat and imagined what that might be like for her, a light bulb flashed, and I shared, "I think maybe when you start giving yourself permission to let go of that loyalty and go after the things you really want, like theater and show choir, then your motivation to work on your dancing technique will skyrocket. What do you think?"

Her eyes lit up.

Derailed by Rejection

My daughter's not the only one who got derailed by life experiences and let them define her. It happened to me too.

Two years after I started my blog, I let rejection take me off the front row, and I quit on myself. Of course, at the time, I called it fate. I let the lack of people's response, a stolen computer, and an expired hosting site let me believe writing wasn't in the cards for me. They were all "signs" from God that it just wasn't meant to be.

Writing was what truly brought me to life after my battle with thyroid cancer; it filled me with purpose and vitality. I felt a rush of excitement whenever I encountered something that sparked my creativity, especially when I could carve out time in a coffee shop to explore those ideas. It had a way of making every space sacred, whether it was the nook in my bedroom or the bleachers in my kid's school auditorium. When I let myself sink in, play with the insight, and craft it into words, heaven descended. Finding the right words to express your inner experience can open you up to a new way of seeing the world. It was play, growth, and something holy all wrapped into one.

I thought surely someone else would benefit from what those musings did for me, so I started sharing them to Facebook friends and family. There were several people who encouraged me and engaged in conversation around the topics, but the crickets I got, more often than not, began drowning that out. Every time I checked back and saw my heartfelt words sitting there unacknowledged, it felt like not getting picked for the kickball team. You know, that feeling of standing there where everyone can see you weren't wanted–that you're not a valuable asset.

It feels like being stabbed in the heart, wanting to hide your wound so no one sees how vulnerable you are. My inner critic saw my hurt and did what it does best: pulled me out of the gymnasium so I wouldn't have to feel the pain of that again. I began writing less frequently and claimed I was too busy, but my work was acting as my defense attorney.

One day, I opened an email that read, "Your site has expired," and my whole body went into a panic. "No! That can't be true!" I searched frantically, trying to log in and find the words I'd birthed into the world, but all my efforts were in vain. Nothing was working to resurrect them. I gave up in defeat, dropped to the floor, and grieved more than I did the day my grandmother passed away–and I loved her a lot. She'd been my biggest cheerleader, affirming me with, "Kate, you have a gift. You should write a book."

Earlier that year, before I let rejection get the best of me, I'd planned to take all my blogs and have them bound, like a baby book that holds all your memories. I wanted it for myself but also thought maybe they'd make nice gifts for people. I cried and cried until I didn't have anything left, then got up and resigned myself to doing something more valuable with my time. Why invest any more energy into something I was never good at anyway? It was time to move on; this was God closing the door.

I redirected my energy and attention back into things I was "good" at: things people acknowledged and wanted me to do, like helping them. I started picking up more hours in the clinic again and took on an interim ministry position at the church. Just like my daughter did that night after she didn't get a callback, I numbed out that desire and "accepted reality." However, that acceptance was more like self-rejection wearing a mask.

Over time, my body began echoing the abandonment and unrest within my soul in the same way my daughter's had that morning. After three years of suppressing my desires and doing what I believed God wanted me to, I finally found the courage to come back home and get honest.

Overcoming Our Past

Past disappointments often shape our beliefs about ourselves and influence the direction of our future. The times when we stood on stage, feeling vulnerable under the watchful gaze of our audience, tended to fuel the self-doubt and sense of inadequacy that were already lurking, waiting to be confirmed. But what if instead of letting them define us, we choose resiliency over resignation?

Retreating in the face of rejection and burying our aspirations under the weight of self-doubt denies us the opportunity to pursue our passions and live authentically. Our inner critic thinks it's keeping us safe, but escaping the sting of rejection is an inside game.

Overcoming our past starts with coming back home to ourselves. When we transform the energy of our inner critic into a cheering grandmother, our dreams get wings. It's never too late to rewrite your story.

GOOD GIRL RX: Transform Your Inner Critic into Your Inner Cheerleader

Breaking free from self-sabotage isn't about avoiding failure or rejection but nurturing a belief in ourselves that withstands the ups and downs. It's choosing to align with our dreams, to transform the voice of self-doubt into one of encouragement, and to reclaim the passions we may have tucked away. Resilience grows every time we choose to stand in self-acceptance rather than letting past disappointments define us. Let this be an invitation to hold yourself with compassion and courage, believing in your ability to take that next step forward.

Reflection Questions:

1. Recall a time when you let go of something you loved due to fear of failure or rejection. How might it feel to revisit this with a renewed sense of belief in yourself?
2. Think about the voice of your inner critic that questions your worth after a setback. What name might you give this voice to recognize when it's speaking? Imagine a more compassionate, supportive voice—what might it say to encourage you instead?
3. Consider this: "What if, instead of staying loyal to something you've outgrown, you began being loyal to yourself?" How could this shift change the way you respond to setbacks or challenges?

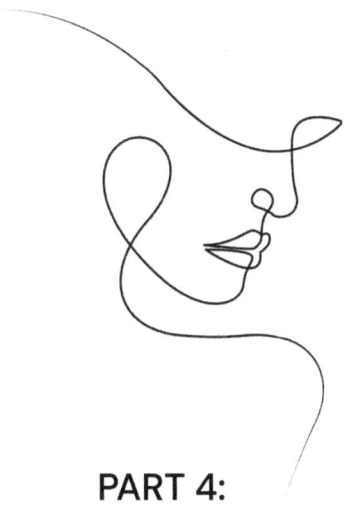

PART 4:

THE GOOD GIRL WHO FOUND HER TRUE SELF

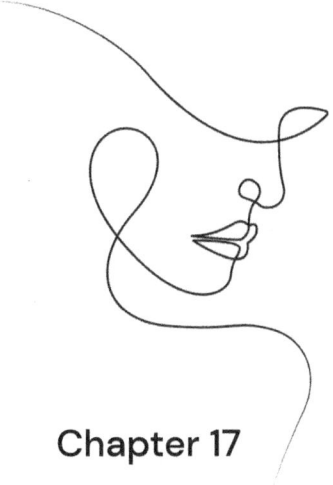

Chapter 17

Lost and Found: Losing Yourself in Relationships

"The greatest gift you can give another person is your own wholeness."
Richard Rohr[35]

It used to get under my skin when I'd come home for a visit after I first got married, and my mom would ask me if I was okay, commenting that I seemed to have lost my confidence. It felt like an attack on my husband and my marriage, which, in my perspective, was amazing. I was truly happy and didn't understand what she was worried about. It annoyed me that she couldn't see things from my perspective, but looking back, I can now see what she was witnessing. As much as I loved being married, in the "leaving and cleaving," I lost myself.

It wasn't anything he or I did intentionally; it just kind of happened. I thought that was a good thing. We were supposed to

---

[35] Themes expressed in Rohr, Richard. *Falling Upward: A Spirituality for the Two Halves of Life.* Jossey-Bass, 2011.

be united, right? He became my best friend, and we did everything together. We made decisions together. We worked through our disagreements together. We were one. Our marriage was a healthy dance of interdependence, except when I shrunk myself in the shadow of his confidence and laid down my aspirations to avoid feeling the risk of disconnection, that is.

My husband never asked or expected that of me, and it wasn't that I didn't do things independently. I had my own interests and often traveled without him. The problem was never about location but my ability to move freely and trust myself when I was with him.

Misplacing Our Identity

When I was alone, I could act in freedom, but in his presence, I struggled with indecision. When he wasn't in the car, I trusted myself, but if he was riding shotgun, I hesitated, as if I needed his approval of my choices. His disagreement and criticism of the route I took or my choice to go to the gas station on the opposite side of the highway were fuel for my insecurity. The more fearful I became of his reactions to my decisions, the more I second-guessed myself, and the more hesitant and indecisive I got, the more annoyed he became. The strategy of trying to guess what he wanted me to do to keep us on the same page became a barricade to him riding in the car with the confident woman he had married. That's what fear does. I was repressing my assertiveness to protect our bond, and instead of growing in my self-assurance, I began losing it.

We don't wake up one day and decide to operate in fear. It's a byproduct of the experiences imprinted in our biology. I had freedom to make my own decisions before I got married; my parents were busy working and managing their own lives. If I wanted something, I had to take initiative and that assertiveness served me well. I did all my college planning on my own, applied for scholarships, filled out the paperwork to receive a Pell Grant, and followed my interest to a private college an older friend was attending. I moved forward, explored my options, and traveled across the country, embracing the things my heart led me to do. That sense of self-trust started dissolving, however, when I vowed before God to become "one" in marriage.

When I came home after work and started trying to share about my day but was met with a lack of interest, I pulled my words back and closed my heart a little. Over time, I stopped sharing, believing my experiences at work were too separate from his world and a source of disconnection. I hated that feeling of not being able to relate or have my excitement mirrored. Those experiences were such a big part of me, and I had so much I wanted to share with him. I mean, he was my best friend. Who else was I going to process all my highs, lows, and insights with?

Every time I tried and was met with silence instead of curiosity, my heart deflated, and that cue of danger was stored in my bank of memories. His lack of engagement not only felt threatening to our unity, it hurt. We were supposed to be one, and his response felt like distance. Every time it happened, I'd start thinking, *maybe I just need to quit this job so I'm not living a different life apart from my husband. I'm supposed to be his helpmate and encourage him in his giftings.* I was afraid that my passions and interests would take us down two different paths and hurt our marriage. I wanted to be a part of what he was a part of; I wanted us to have shared experiences. I wanted us to feel connected, and it felt like an either/or: either I stayed at the job I loved and compartmentalized that part of my life, or I could quit or cut back my hours so my heart wasn't so invested and be obedient to my purpose of helping my husband. I thought being united meant there was no division between us. I didn't understand the difference between unity and enmeshment.

I was so afraid of losing what I valued and feeling that sting of rejection that I gave up the parts of myself that might contribute to that. I equated not asking about my day with not caring about me, and that hurt too much. If I didn't do things he wasn't interested in, then I didn't have to face feeling hurt when he didn't ask about them. Instead of working through that insecurity, I opted to repress my self-expression and abandoned my passions.

Coming Face to Face with My Habit of Self-Abandonment

One day, while walking up the hill in my neighborhood, listening to an audio recording of my mastery coaching lesson through my airpods, I heard my instructor say something that made me rewind and replay the track. She was explaining different kinds of impaired birthrights that impact our ability to move forward toward change and growth. One of them ignited a lightbulb of clarity within me: "All children have the right to *be separate but still belong...*"

I had that impaired birthright! I'd lost the ability to individuate myself and take confident action without being afraid I'd lose that deep connection I needed and craved. That "right to take action" and separate ourselves from others is learned between six and twelve months when a child starts crawling and exploring their world in the context of secure attachment. I may have felt safe enough to separate from my parents, but for some reason, I didn't feel that same security with my husband. I think it was because the risk felt greater—there was more to lose.

I came face to face with my lost sense of self as my children started graduating and my health started declining. I finally started reconnecting with who I was apart from others again. I started reclaiming my birthright to be separate and connected at the same time. I started expressing myself more and teaching my husband what I needed. I started believing he loved and cared about me, even if he struggled to articulate it. I stopped determining what I should and shouldn't be doing based on someone else's response, or lack thereof, and my marriage and confidence began to flourish. It took a lot of trial and error, tears, screaming, and painful navigating to get there, but moving courageously through the tension of reclaiming a strong sense of self was one of the best things I've ever done. It was a necessary and vital part of my healing journey.

This same belief affected my business for a long time. I had an underlying fear that growing my business would prevent me from sharing experiences with my husband in retirement. My business coach called this out one day and asked, "What if the opposite is true? What if moving forward into the things God is calling you to do opens the doorway for opportunities for your husband? What if God is waiting for you to do what you already know to do and your hesitation to move forward until your husband finds his path and passions is the very thing blocking him from discovering his own?"

That landed. I was holding back in a codependent pattern, wanting to make sure he was happy before I'd allow myself to be. It was an invitation to come back home to the confidence and exploration I embodied as a young college student. My husband didn't need or even ask me to shrink myself for him. Love never asks that of us.

Wholeness: The Foundation for True Connection

Shrinking and holding ourselves back doesn't build bridges of connection; it creates dams. We repress our authentic selves when we hold back, give up, or stop pursuing the things that inspire us because we fear losing our sense of belonging. This prevents us from being truly known and hinders the most valuable contribution we can make to our relationships: our wholeness. We may stay relationally safe, but our true self is lost along the way. There is no win in that equation. True unity is not achieved by limiting our individuality, but by bringing the fullness of it into our relationships! When you come back home to the truth of who you are, you discover that wholeness is the foundation for the deeper connection your heart has been craving.

Losing Parts of Myself to Become Whole

It took losing my thyroid, both of my ovaries, and my sanity to finally break free from the habits that were contributing to recurring health and relational challenges and keeping me from moving forward in life. Transforming our health, our relationships, and our lives is always a continual process of letting go: letting go of old ways of being that aren't serving us anymore. As C. Everett Koop said, *"True healing is the restoration of the person to wholeness, not the removal of symptoms."*[36]

I spent so long trying to *fix* myself by addressing the symptoms, but what I came to understand is that healing didn't come by focusing on what was broken. It came when I started addressing the deeper roots of self-abandonment, shame, and fear. Healing happened when I stopped sacrificing parts of myself and began the work of wholeness—restoring who I was created to be.

Ephesians 4:22-23 (MSG) speaks to this truth: "Everything— and I do mean everything—connected with that old way of life has to go. It's rotten through and through. Get rid of it! And then take on an entirely new way of life—a God-fashioned life, a life renewed from the inside."

We often get this confused and think denying ourselves means denying our needs and desires, but what I have finally come to understand is that God was never asking me to sacrifice my true self. He wanted me to break free from my adapted self! The call to deny is the call to surrender our appeasing, pleasing,

---

36 Koop, C. Everett. *Whatever Happened to the Human Race?* Revell, 1983.

and protective strategies that are blocking us from all He wants for us. When we start loosening our identification with our personas and start allowing our true self in Christ to emerge, we find ourselves. We come back home to the truth of who we are: the *Imago Dei*. When we find the courage to let our old ways of being go, we find the freedom and confidence we've been looking for all along.

Redefining Self

In Internal Family Systems (IFS), a therapeutic model developed by Dr. Richard Schwartz, the *Self* is defined as the unchanging, grounded center of who we truly are. Unlike the parts of us that carry burdens, fears, and adapted survival strategies, the Self is inherently whole. It is characterized by what Schwartz calls the "8 Cs"—compassion, curiosity, calm, clarity, confidence, courage, creativity, and connectedness.[37]

Dr. Alison Cook, co-author of *Boundaries for Your Soul*, explains that our *true self*—the God-reflecting center of who we are—has been covered up by protective parts that take on roles to keep us safe, loved, and accepted.[38] These parts may look like over-achieving, pleasing, perfecting, or hiding, but they are not the essence of who we are. They are strategies we've adopted in response to fear, shame, or pain. When we confuse these protective strategies with our true selves, we disconnect from the Spirit of Love within us. Instead of reflecting God's image, we reflect our adaptations—our striving, our people-pleasing, our need to prove our worth.

The biblical definition of self aligns beautifully with this. Scripture doesn't call us to deny the *true self*—the one created

---

37   Schwartz, Richard C. *Internal Family Systems Therapy*. Guilford Press, 1995.
38   Cook, Alison, and Kimberly Miller. *Boundaries for Your Soul: How to Turn Your Overwhelming Thoughts and Feelings into Your Greatest Allies*. Thomas Nelson, 2018.

in God's image. It calls us to lay down the *false self*, shaped by ego and fear, to uncover the new self that is alive in Christ. Paul describes this in Colossians 3:9-10 (ESV): "Do not lie to one another, seeing that you have put off the old self with its practices and have put on the new self, which is being renewed in knowledge after the image of its creator." As we untangle from these outdated patterns, we find the very life they were working so hard to protect. We are renewed, like an antique chair restored to its original glory.

Breaking Down to Break Through

As humans, we balk at changing until things get so bad and uncomfortable that we can no longer go on with business as usual. We wait for crisis, trauma, loss, disease, and tragedy before we get down to looking at who we are, what we are doing, how we are living, what we are feeling, and what we are believing in order to embrace change.

When I first started my coaching business, I looked at my husband and said, *"I think it's going to take a crisis before these women are ready to invest in change."* It made me sad. I wanted to spare them what I had gone through and rescue them from it, but I've come to realize it's in the loss that we become ready to be found. The discomfort has to get intense enough for us to be ready to navigate the fear of letting go of our old ways of being. We don't like uncertainty. We'd rather know who we are and what we're supposed to be doing than break free from our attachment to a life that is crippling. We cling to the familiar, resist change, and project our past onto our future; our need for certainty and grip on familiarity enslaves us to our present realities and the narratives defining them. We may feel like we're going crazy and coming unglued, but those moments are the gateways to our breakthroughs. It's in the coming apart that we are recreated and the letting go of old beliefs and programming that we are freed.

Joe Dispena, author of *Breaking the Habit of Being Yourself*, states, "The greatest habit you can ever break is the habit of being yourself."[39] Falling apart is the catalyst to shedding the personas we've carefully constructed to stay safe, accepted, or seen as 'good. These breakdowns create fertile ground for growth and authenticity, allowing our true selves to emerge.

Transformation always involves a shedding. Just as a butterfly must struggle to break free from its chrysalis, a snake to shed its skin, and a baby to outgrow the safety of the womb, we, too, must push through resistance to shed our old selves. This necessary pain leads to growth, renewal, and the emergence of our truest, most resilient selves. It's like the man at the pool of Bethesda (John 5:6, ESV). When Jesus asked, 'Do you want to be well?' The man could only see the reasons he couldn't reach the pool. His illness had become so familiar, so much a part of his identity, that he struggled to step into the unknown. Like him, we can cling to the safety of what we know, even when it's keeping us stuck. But real change begins when we're willing to face the discomfort of letting go—of old identities, patterns, and ways of being—so something new can emerge.

While I genuinely wish to protect other women from hardship and educate them to avoid my experiences, I am finally coming to terms with the importance of these challenges. They served as a crucial catalyst for me, teaching me valuable lessons that helped me learn to let go of my old ways of being. Love is not a rescuing energy but one that allows people the space to learn and grow. It witnesses, shows compassion, and holds them within it, offering safety and shelter without trying to fix them or remove the experiences that shape their growth. No wonder we get so mad at God for not answering our prayers for protection. He's

---

39 Dispenza, Joe. *Breaking the Habit of Being Yourself: How to Lose Your Mind and Create a New One*. Hay House, 2012.

not doing what we would do. We are confusing love with fear, viewing it as a rescuing energy rather than an embracing one.

God never asked us to sacrifice our true selves. He invites us to surrender the false self—our striving, our fear, our need to prove ourselves—and come home to the truth of who we already are: whole, loved, and made to reflect Him. In letting go, we don't lose ourselves; we finally find ourselves.

GOOD GIRL RX: Restore a Strong Sense of Self

Rediscovering yourself is a journey back to wholeness—a gradual process of reconnecting with the parts of you that have always been there, even if they've been quieted or tucked away. Allow yourself the grace to explore and reclaim these pieces. Trust that in finding yourself, you are not losing connection to God or others but enhancing it. True unity and belonging come from bringing the fullness of who you are into your relationships.

Reflection Questions:

1. Reflect on the Biblical idea of self-denial presented in this chapter. How have you confused denying your true self with denying your false self or personas? How does that distinction feel in your body?
2. In what ways have you lost a part of your true self in relationships, work, or life transitions? Can you think of a specific moment or pattern where you began to shrink or suppress your individuality?
3. Reflect on the idea that being unified in a relationship doesn't mean losing yourself. How might you begin to reclaim your sense of individuality while still feeling connected to the people you love?

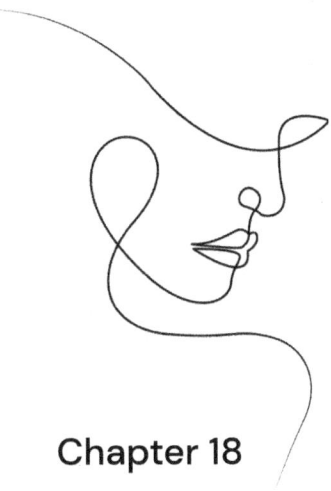

Chapter 18

Getting Unshackled From Shame

> *"If you want short-term obedience, scare or shame people. If you want transformation, anchor them to God's unconditional love."*
> Jonathan Merritt

Shame is the thing I see that shackles so many women and used to have a fierce hold on me. It can still sneak up, grab me by the hair, and pull me back when I perceive that what I'm doing might not be okay for someone else. It grips me hardest when I dare to voice my own desires, feeling guilty for even wanting them. It tightens its hold when I sense my needs might inconvenience others or overshadow their own. Suddenly, I'm engulfed in self-criticism, chastising myself for not living up to some standard of respectability. I can always tell when it's taken me out by the posture I find myself in. Shame lowers our chin, averts our eyes, drops our shoulders, and sinks us into a posture of defeat. It takes us into closets, cars, and under covers to hide us and says, *"Don't look at me. I'm flawed."*

Wrestling with Guilt in the Church Pew

I sat in the pews of the First Baptist Church watching my daughter's all city choir concert; only I wasn't really watching; I was wrestling. There was a war going on inside of me and no matter how hard I tried to attend to the voices in front of me, the shouts of my soul were drowning them out.

It all started that morning.

The Trigger: The Budget and the Hair Appointment

My husband had asked me to come into the office to review the budget and help figure out how to cover my daughter's dance fees. As I scanned the numbers, my phone buzzed—a reminder for the hair appointment I'd scheduled for the next day. The prompt for confirmation started tugging at my guilt strings. I hadn't told him about it, and I knew there was no money set aside. Then later, my daughter hit me with, "Why don't we ever have any money? Shouldn't we have more now that I'm the only one left at home?" How could I explain? I was working more back then. I'm trying to grow my business and am investing a lot in training and writing this book... and honestly, I know we had more back then, but I don't want to go back to the stress I was carrying before.

That's when the storm started brewing. Guilt stepped in and began its assault:

- *"How can you sit here and not do more to help your family?"*
- *"You shouldn't have invested in this book—you should've waited until she was in college."*
- *"That choice was so selfish. You need to fix this."*

The Shame Spiral

Later that night, as I sat beside my husband in the church, with time to spare before the concert began, I tried letting him in. I told him how much I wanted to be generous and hated that I wasn't contributing more right now. I hoped that saying it out loud might release some of the heaviness, that his reassurance might pull me out from under the shame that was draped over me like a weighted blanket. Instead, his response landed like a no-nonsense lesson in cause and effect. "Well, get ready because Christmas is right around the corner."

The dagger of guilt that was already in my chest twisted and spiraled into seething shame. I know he didn't mean to hurt me. I think he was feeling the pressure, too—trying to meet me in my reality. But instead of reassurance, I felt like he was agreeing with my inner critic. *You should feel guilty. You're not doing enough. You're hurting your family.*

That voice of self-blame jumped on that cue and grew louder. *I'm so angry you said yes to writing this book. You funneled all the money toward yourself and put your family in this place of scarcity... again. You're selfish. If you really cared, you'd get a real job and work hard like other moms.*

As I sat there under the weight of those condemning words, I felt myself go numb—floating away to avoid the impact, like some part of me was trying to protect itself by shutting down. I knew what was happening. I've worked hard to recognize these storms when they hit, and I tried to use the tools I've learned to ground myself. I scanned for cues of safety, anchoring my gaze on the organ pipes, the stained-glass windows, anything that might pull me back to the present moment. I shifted my focus to my body, feeling the pressure of the floor under my feet, willing myself to settle. But my husband, probably noticing that I'd left the building, started trying to engage me by making lighthearted jokes. Instead, it deepened my frustration and pissed me off that he was clueless to what I was feeling. I didn't want to be cheered up. I didn't need lightness. I needed someone to see me—to see the storm, the shame, the fight going on inside of me. If I could have found the voice to say it, I would have whispered: *Please help me get out from under this shame. It's about to take me out.*

The Deeper Work: Journaling Through the Storm

It wasn't just about the hair appointment. It wasn't even about the budget. The real conflict was inside me. One part of me wanted to care for myself, to honor something I'd looked forward to—a simple hair appointment the week of my birthday. But another part, my inner critic, shamed me for it. It called me selfish and uncaring, accusing me of letting my family down. Before I knew it, I was typing a text message telling my hair stylist I needed to cancel and then reprimanding myself for feeling sad afterward. *Kate, you chose this. You said yes to investing in this book. That yes came with a lot of no's. You're a grown woman—this was your decision.* It worked for a moment, and I shifted my focus to gratitude, but the funk was still there, hanging over me. Realizing I was in no condition to be productive that morning, I reached for my journal to get curious.

The Process: Thoughts, Emotions, and Memories

I wrote *I don't have enough money to get my hair done. I had to cancel my appointment the week of my birthday. There's not enough for the things I want and need. I'm feeling sad, hurt, and like I matter less.* Next, I scanned my feelings wheel and landed on *inadequate*. That was it. *There's not enough for the things I want and need... and for the people I love. I have to give up what I need so they have enough.*

As soon as I named it, something began to shift. The weighted blanket took on energy and started swirling inside of me, stirring up memories and emotions from the past, building in intensity until it morphed into an F5 tornado. As I focused on the felt sense in my body, a vivid memory surfaced: the night I sat in my apartment closet, overwhelmed with the inability to protect my daughter from having to transfer schools and feeling utterly powerless to meet her needs. In that moment of despair, I'd banged my head against the wall, consumed by thoughts of self-harm. It felt like a bear standing up on its hind feet, poised to attack, but the target of its rage was me.

The Realization: Shame as a Protector

The next morning, as I processed this memory through tears, I started to see what my harsh inner critic wanted for me. It was using shame to try and motivate me—to push me into fixing the problem so I wouldn't have to feel inadequate. It was saying *If I can get you to do more—get a job, work harder—you won't have to feel like you're not enough. If I can make you see how your choices hurt your family, you'll never let it happen again.*

That anxious, angry energy wasn't trying to destroy me. It was trying to protect me—from feeling like I was failing everyone. But the truth is: toxic shame doesn't protect. It entraps us-keeping us stuck in a cycle of never-enough.

The Path Forward

Guilt and shame often come with good intentions. At their core, they're trying to keep us safe, aligned with what we value, and connected to others. But they're driven by fear and fear rarely leads us toward true growth. Instead, it traps us in survival mode—clouding our perspective, warping our reality, and whispering lies about our worth.

Toxic shame tells us: *You're not enough. You're selfish. You're failing.* It feels like the truth at the moment, but shame isn't a reliable guide. It doesn't point us toward change or freedom—it shuts us down. When we're caught in shame's grip, all we see are cues of danger that confirm our greatest fears. In my case, the storm of shame told me I was hurting my family when the opposite was true. Staying in my yes—honoring the call to write this book—wasn't abandoning them. It was an act of deep faith and courage, a trust that this work would grow me and, in time, ripple out to bless my family and the world.

The Cost of Staying Stuck

Shame sabotages its own intention. It pushes us to do more, be more, and prove our worth, but the pressure it creates wreaks havoc on our minds and bodies. The chronic stress of toxic shame triggers a biological stress response—flooding us with cortisol, weakening our immune systems, and driving anxiety, depression, and self-sabotage.[40] It keeps us stuck in cycles of over-giving, perfectionism, and self-criticism that derail our health, steal our joy, and rob our families of our presence. The truth is shame doesn't help us live better lives. It constricts us. It silences us. It stops us from stepping into the fullness of who we are.

The Antidote to Shame: Love

If shame locks us in fear, love is the key that sets us free. Love doesn't need to shame us into change; it invites us into transformation. When we anchor ourselves in love—when we allow ourselves to be seen and held in our wholeness—it changes everything. Love quiets the critical voice. It softens the tension. It dissolves fear and makes space for healing, peace, and the restoration of our true selves.

Jesus modeled this so beautifully. He didn't shame people into following him. He called them out of their hiding and into connection. He saw their hearts, their struggles, their worth and

---

40 Fishkin, Gerald Loren. *The Science of Shame and Its Treatment*. Praeger, 2016.

invited them to walk in freedom. That's the same invitation we have today: to trade shame for self-compassion, to release the weight we carry, and to walk with love as our guide.

GOOD GIRL RX: Trade Shame for Self-Love

Shame may push us to act, but it keeps us trapped in cycles of stress and self-sabotage. To break free, we need to pause, investigate shame's intention, and update the strategy. When we replace shame's voice with self-compassion and align ourselves with God's heart, we can step into the grounding, liberating energy of love.

From this place, we don't just heal. We become our truest, most fruitful selves. And when we live from that fullness, we don't just set ourselves free—we show others what's possible.

Reflection Questions:

1. Think of the last time you felt inadequate or judged yourself for not doing enough.
    - What triggered those feelings? What did you see, hear, or sense that spiraled you into self-reproach?
2. What thoughts and emotions came up for you? What did that feel like in your body?
3. What did you need to hear at that moment? If you feel blocked, ask yourself: What would I say to someone I love who was feeling this way?

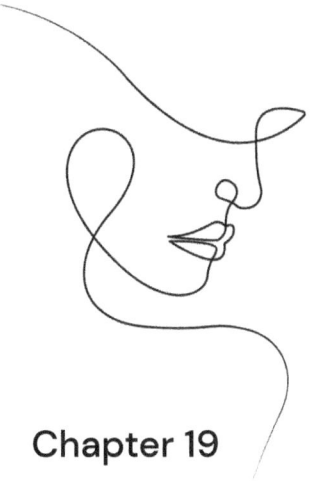

Chapter 19

Beyond Labels: Recognizing the Good in All of Us

"Sin is not the primary thing that is true about us. Before we are anything else, we are made in God's image, and we are made to reflect that image in the way we live. Before scripture tells us anything else about ourselves, it tells us we are good. I think that's because that's the way God intended it. When we ground ourselves in the fact that God created us good, we are capable of confronting all the other things that are true about us, even the difficult things. Love is tremendously healing."
Danielle Shroyer, author of Original Blessing

Brenda's Story

I sat across the screen from a young mom recently and asked her what emotion she was checking in with. She answered, "Well, it's been a rough morning. My son had a meltdown in the kitchen because he couldn't figure out what he wanted for breakfast and nothing I suggested was helping. I couldn't fix it for him. I felt torn again between what my other kids needed from me and needing to get everyone fed and out the door. My husband was able to come in and give him a hug while I was tending to the other two. That calmed him down, and he was good after that. I'm learning he doesn't need me to help him or fix it. He just needs a hug, for me to be there with him. But when he starts crying and screaming it just makes me want to pull back; it shuts me down."

We talked through what was happening in her body when that was going on and the emotions, unmet need, and stories attached. "I just need them not to scream. I need them to be happy. I don't want them to feel left out or unloved. I don't like feeling like I am putting them off. It makes me feel guilty. I always feel so torn. I can't figure out where I'm supposed to be and what my responsibility is, and it ramps up my anxiety. If I attend to one of them, the other could get mad that I am not spending time with them. I feel so torn, and I have to go make them feel better."

As we dug into the story lurking beneath her experience, we found this narrative: *If my kids are unhappy, I must not be a good mom. I'm not doing a good enough job. I'm not enough.*

" I want to be a good mom and do a good job. If I was, I would feel proud of myself and them. I'd feel good, and then I'd want to keep doing things for them. I wish I could feel like this more."

As we loaded up what that would feel like in her body, she shared, "The heaviness is gone. I can smile and laugh more easily and not be so upright. When I'm feeling this way, I can interact with them, be silly, and I'm not pulling back in avoidance and getting on my phone. I have more compassion and can help them figure out what needs to be met. I'm able to be there for my kids. It feels like... presence."

Next, I asked, "What would someone have to believe to be feeling that way and able to just relax?"

"That they're a good mom," she replied.

"What are you believing right now?"

"I'm a good mom."

She sent me this text the next day: "My son had another massive meltdown in the car on the way to school this morning. Remembering what we talked about yesterday, though, I was able to breathe through it, reciting my mantra: *I am a good mom. I am patient. I am loving. I am kind,* so that I could get us all safely to school. As we arrived at the school, he was still screaming, crying, and refusing to let me help. So, I took my daughter in and was able to let go of the necessity for him to be on time for school. I came back to the car and was able to sit with him and hold him until he felt better. We went home so I could drop off my youngest son so he could eat breakfast and so my other son could get a hug from his dad. Then the two of us went back to school, and he happily went in. I was able to let go of the story that he had to be at school on time and remember that he's only six and that in that moment, what he needed most was me. Seriously. Thank you."

Do you see where we get off track? We are basing our self-perception on what we sense in the world around us. If someone cries, screams, stomps their feet, or gets mad, our entire body senses their dis-ease and brings to mind all the implicit memories of when we've felt that way before and how bad we felt about ourselves. *I must be doing something wrong. They're not pleased with me. It must be my fault they're so unhappy.* So we make a decision to do whatever it takes to never feel that way again! Feeling bad feels like shame and who wants to feel that? In an effort to avoid the shame, guilt, anxiety, or whatever emotion arises when others are expressing displeasure, anger, frustration, agitation, make sure to do something to alleviate that. If we can alleviate it, then we can stop feeling so bad and start feeling good again.

Making their actions and reactions mean something about us gives us a sense of control. If we internalize it and blame ourselves, then we can do something about it. We have a way of restoring that sense of connectedness and safety we need. If it's not about us, then it feels out of our control. We feel helpless, and that never feels safe. So, in an effort to restore a sense of safety, we assume responsibility and reclaim a sense of power by taking it on ourselves, but man, does that get heavy and burdensome over time! What we thought would help us to feel good again actually serves to fuel anxiety, overwhelm, depression, and chronic illness.

These things don't develop out of security but out of our belief that others' discomfort is evidence of our inadequacy. We start equating other's pleasure with a sense of peace, and as soon as someone stubs a toe, we lose it–literally. *Crap, here we go again. I've got a crying, whiny child that needs my attention, and there is not enough of me to go around. Lord, help me.*

Are you seeing the problem here?

What if it was okay for them to stub their toe and cry? What if it wasn't our responsibility to ensure that they're always happy? What if being a good mom is actually more about believing we are loved even when others are upset and that our acceptance doesn't hinge on their response? What difference might that make in our lives? In the lives of our children? What might be the impact?

Goodness Is Who You Are

If there's one thing I've learned from my work with women—having a front-row seat with God to witness the depths of their souls—it's that at their core, they are pure love, beauty, and light. Beneath the overwhelm, anxiety, lashing out, avoidance, and self-criticism lies a little girl who longs to feel loved and extend that love back into the world. *Goodness is who she is, and it's who you are.*

You were made in the image of the Divine. That means goodness isn't something you earn or achieve; it's your birthright. It's the sacred truth of who you've always been. But over time, that truth gets buried. Somewhere along the way, you may have received the message that you weren't enough just as you are—feeding deep insecurity and stripping away your freedom to show up as your true self. So you adapted. You learned what you needed to do to survive, to stay safely connected to love, and to have your basic needs met.

And it worked. If you're reading this, you made it. You stayed safe. But those adaptations—those protective strategies—came at a cost. They hid the real you. They convinced you to judge yourself harshly when you lashed out or shut down. They told you that something was wrong with you when, in truth, they were just trying to protect the sacred within you.

Coming Out of Hiding

The souls of so many little girls received the message that they weren't good enough just as they are, feeding deep insecurity and stripping away their freedom to be themselves. They adapted to survive, learning how to stay safely connected to love and have their basic needs met. If you're reading this, you made it. You survived. You stayed safe. But now, it's time to come out of hiding. It's time to slowly emerge from the cocoon of your adaptations, break free from the patterns that once protected you, and find the safety to unfold those wings so you can fly. And it's okay to move slowly. I know your nervous system's need for safety. This isn't about rushing. It's about remembering the truth of who you are.

And that's where *how we see ourselves* becomes so important.

When we view ourselves through a lens of lack, we look at behaviors—our own and others'—and make quick judgments. We isolate. We blame. We shame. We see a woman who's overwhelmed and think, *She's failing.* We see a "codependent" and think, *She's needy.* We see a "narcissist" and think, *He's a monster.* But what if we looked deeper? What if we chose to see ourselves and others the way God sees us—beyond behavior, beyond masks, straight to the heart?

Danielle Shroyer, author of Original Blessing, explains this beautifully. The message of the book is that the deepest truth of the world is that we find our home in God because God is our home."[41] This truth changes everything. It shifts the lens. It softens the edges. It invites us to trade judgment for compassion, shame for love, and fear for safety. Because when we *know* we are inherently loved, inherently good, and inherently whole, we can finally stop hiding.

You don't have to keep proving yourself. You don't have to stay in survival mode. It's safe to come out of hiding and trust the truth of who you are.

Correcting the Lens in Which We See Ourselves

So how did we get here? How did we lose sight of this truth—that we are inherently good, loved, and whole?

Jonathan Merritt, a writer on faith and culture, explores this in his interview with Danielle Shroyer. He explains:

"The doctrine of 'original sin' asserts that human nature was corrupted due to the first sin by Adam and Eve and, therefore, all humans are inherently sinful. It's a 'theological construct,' which means it isn't explicitly laid out in the Christian scriptures, but rather derives from quilting together various passages."[42]

This perspective began to take root with Augustine in the 4th Century AD and gained widespread acceptance during the

---

41 Shroyer, Danielle. *Original Blessing: Putting Sin in Its Rightful Place*. Fortress Press, 2016.
42 Merritt, Jonathan. "Author: Jesus Didn't Believe In 'Original Sin' And Neither Should We." *Religion News Service*, 13 Jan. 2017, https://religionnews.com/2017/01/13/author-jesus-didnt-believe-in-original-sin-and-neither-should-we/.

Reformation. Merritt explains that while the early church viewed sin as an action or even an illness, Augustine introduced the idea of an inborn sin nature. Suddenly, human bodies—our "flesh"—became suspect. Salvation became about sin management.

And while this framework may have offered structure, it also planted a seed of shame that continues to sprout today, especially in women. Danielle Shroyer offers a different perspective:

"People know they sin. What they don't know is what to do about it. I don't think the best answer is admitting you are irrevocably bad. I think it's realizing your home has been in God all along, and it's time you head that direction, because abundant life is waiting."

Do you feel the difference?

This isn't about dismissing sin or excusing harmful behaviors. It's about shifting from shame to love. From disconnection to reconnection. From believing we are "bad" to remembering that we are inherently good, created for love, and deeply worthy. Yes, we fall short. Yes, we act in fear, scarcity, and self-protection. Yes, we hurt ourselves and others. But that doesn't make us inherently bad. It makes us human. And being human? That's not an accident. God didn't make a mistake when He designed us with the capacity for fear, self-protection, or dissociation. These are survival tools—gifts woven into our nervous system so we can stay alive in our human bodies. Without fear and self-preservation, we wouldn't survive in the face of real threat. Without the ability to dissociate, we'd be overwhelmed and consumed by the weight of our traumas.

These patterns, though imperfect, are part of the divine design that allows us to keep going, to keep breathing, to keep living. They are not evidence of our brokenness but of our resilience. And when we can respect and appreciate this design, we can begin to align and abide within it—learning to move beyond survival into a place of safety, connection, and healing.

When we see ourselves through God's eyes—when we look past the behaviors and into the heart—we find a new lens. We remember who we truly are:

> "God saw all that he had made, and it was very good... (Genesis 1:31).

God declared you good simply by existing. Before you did anything—before you were productive or helpful or kind—He looked at you and said, "It was very good." That goodness isn't something you achieve. It's who you are.

"We have spent centuries trying to solve the 'problem' that we're told is at the heart of our humanity. But when we start with a problem, we tend never to get beyond that very mindset."[43]

You were never meant to live in the shadows of shame. The invitation of Jesus is not to shrink into smaller versions of ourselves but to expand—to trade the fear of separation for the joy of connection.

Beyond Behaviors

I caught myself recently as I contemplated sending a message to my friend to see if she would mind if I brought my daughter and a few of her friends to enjoy their lake house for an end-of-the-school-year celebration. I caught myself rehearsing the inner dialogue: *It would just be two friends, and they're both good girls.* I guess what I was implying is, *You won't have to worry about them. They're going to respect your property. They won't be drinking or doing anything 'bad.'*

I find it interesting how strong that label is in my vocabulary and my way of viewing the world. If you're polite, say *"please*

---

43 Merritt, Jonathan. "Author: Jesus Didn't Believe in 'Original Sin' and Neither Should We." *Jonathan Merritt*, 25 Jan. 2017, https://www.jonathanmerritt.com/article/author-jesus-didnt-believe-original-sin-neither.

and thank you," are respectful of my home, don't drink, do drugs, or have sex before marriage, if you hold the door open, pick up someone's book if they drop it, read your Bible in the morning, volunteer to do things without being asked, and help your mom when she looks like she could use it, then you are a *"Good Girl."*

But forget to say thanks, leave your dishes on the table, go to a party without telling your parents and drink a beer, dress too immodestly, have sex before you're married, be too preoccupied with your own stuff to notice when someone drops a book, rush through a doorway without considering who might be behind you—thinking only of yourself and where you're trying to go— have no motivation to read your Bible, don't attend every youth event at your church, and are so focused on your own activities that you never volunteer or lend a helping hand to your mom, then *sorry to inform you,* but you're likely going to be labeled as *"bad."*

Okay, maybe a 'Good Girl' would never call you that, but she is thinking, *Don't ever be like that. How rude. How self-absorbed. How insecure you must be to need alcohol or to dress like that. How mixed up are your priorities to not be starting the day in the Word? How uncaring to walk past others without any regard to their needs. I'll pray for you.* Lots and lots of inward labeling. Lots of noticing. Lots of seeing something she was taught to view as wrong and frowned upon.

I don't say all this to encourage girls to do the latter description but to shed light on what is happening below the surface of the former and what both of these girls have in common: the need to belong and feel safe and secure in their relationships. One is trying to get it from their parents, other adults, and God, while the other from her peers. Neither is good or bad, but simply using a different strategy for meeting her inherent needs. *Oh, if we would only see we're all more alike than different and that every behavior has a positive intention.* What if, like God, we could see beyond behaviors to the good in everyone? What if we stopped labeling each other—and ourselves?

The "Good Girl" may receive smiles, affirmation, and letters of recommendation, but the "Bad Girl" enjoys self-expression and the confidence to set boundaries around her time and energy. She feels comfortable in her own body, has no fear of what people think, and gets what she wants and where she wants, unhinged from needing validation for anything. She has the freedom to scream and cry and shout what she thinks for the world to hear and explore and try new things. I don't know about you, but I'd love a little more of her "could care less" attitude sometimes.

We're All More Alike Than We Realize

I once asked a group of women if they related to being a "Good Girl" growing up. Most said a resounding yes, but their answers revealed so much more:

- "I was the teacher's pet."
- "Yep. I was the charming good girl who all the adults loved and befriended."
- "Well, I tried at first, but I was never good enough, so I quit trying and became a bad girl."
- "I was a good girl but could have an attitude and a sassy mouth; a bit of wild hair too, but mostly good."
- "I was, but I also snuck out and did a lot of things I wasn't supposed to because my mom assumed I was 'fine.'"
- "I did sneaky stuff, too, but no one ever assumed I would do it because I was the good girl."
- "I just was never as bad as my friends."
- "Nope, but I was always asked, 'Why can't you be a good girl?!'" "I tried, but it wasn't considered 'good' enough. I was overly compared to my sister, so I ended up rebelling due to the family/house rules that didn't make sense

and were hypocritical. Then I was labeled 'the problem child.'"
- "Yes and no. My mom was narcissistic, so she made me out to be the bad girl even though everything I did was filling the 'good girl' role. Finally, in high school, I decided to start following the path she was accusing me of."
- "I gave up trying to be good because I couldn't win."

Here's the thing: whether you were the "good girl" or the "bad girl," your core need was the same. To be seen. To be loved. To feel enough. We either swing to the right and proceed with caution, or we realize no matter how much we try, we're going to fall short and be judged, so we give up. That's when the "bad girl" comes out to play. Both strategies are rooted in self-preservation. Neither reflects your true self. Your true self is the carefree little girl, full of creativity, self-expression, goodness, and authentic confidence. She's not loud, but she's bold. She's not shy, but she's graceful. She is both gentle and fierce. She can be soft yet unshakable.

You are not a goody-two-shoes, a bad girl, a people pleaser, a rebel, a slut, or a codependent. You are none of these labels—those are just the masks we wear to protect the tender, sacred parts of ourselves. Sometimes, your true self is quiet, reflecting deeply. Other times, she is unafraid to take up space and let her voice be heard. Sometimes, she moves through life with a fierce determination; other times, she surrenders to the flow and trusts the process. Whether you choose to dress modestly or walk in a string bikini, whether you're dancing wildly in the rain or sitting still in prayer, the important question is not what's "good" or "bad," but what's underlying your actions? Are you aligned with love, authenticity, and freedom—or hiding behind the armor of protection? Your true self doesn't need to prove anything or apologize for existing. She is deeply grounded, rooted in truth, and free to embrace the fullness of life with open-hearted courage.

It's Not What You Do, It's Who You Are

Sometimes, walking on the beach in a sweatshirt and messy bun is a victory. Sometimes, wearing a string bikini without shame is the victory. It's not about what you wear or how you act—it's about *who you're being* and *what you're believing about yourself* as you do it. Are you embodying your true self? Or are you letting the "good" or "bad" girl come out to play to keep you safe?

We all hide in different ways—through people-pleasing, rebellion, shame, or perfectionism. But these are just protective strategies, not who we truly are. God doesn't see the "good girl" or the "bad girl." He sees the profound loss of self and the beauty of who you are underneath. Wouldn't it be amazing if the woman in the burka and the woman in the bikini could sit down together for tea and feel equally free? Truly free?

Here's the check-in:
- What's happening in your body? Is the energy one of love or fear? Constriction or openness?
- Are you aligned with the energy of love, or are you covering up?

The "Good Girl" and the "Bad Girl" are two sides of the same coin, both responding to trauma in different ways—one through fawning and the other through fight. God sees both as a profound loss: a loss of self, a loss of wholeness, and a loss of the unique beauty and truth of who you are. Instead of judging each other, imagine if we could learn from each other and integrate these parts. What if we could resurrect what has been repressed into the shadows and come home to our true selves? That is restoration. That is healing. That is when all of heaven rejoices and jumps up and down.

GOOD GIRL RX: Embody Your Inherent Worth

It's easy to tie our worth to what's happening around us—to the approval of others, the success of our children, or the recognition we receive. But at our core, our worth isn't conditional. It's not something we earn; it's something we embody simply by existing. You are worthy, not because of what you do or give, but because you're here. Breathe that in and rest in that today.

Reflection Questions:

1. Brenda believed that if her kids weren't happy, it meant she wasn't a good mom. What similar stories or beliefs do you hold about your worth? How do they play out in your day-to-day life? How might your experience shift if you let go of those stories and embraced the truth- that your worth is not something that needs validation?
2. Reflect on this idea: "We aren't talking about 'sin nature' but 'human nature.'" How does this shift in perspective affect the way you see yourself and your worth? What might change if you started with the belief that you are inherently good rather than flawed or broken?
3. "Good Girl" or "Bad Girl"—both are ways we protect ourselves. Can you think of a time when you were labeled (or labeled someone else) as "good" or "bad"? How did that label affect the way you saw yourself or them? How might it feel to let go of the labels and focus on the shared desire for love and acceptance?
4. What parts of your true self—boldness, creativity, confidence—feel hidden or repressed? What would it look like to begin reclaiming them?

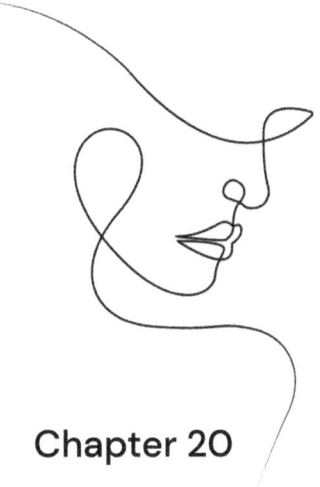

Chapter 20

Getting to Know and Embracing Her Shadow

"Sometimes it is the shadow part that saves our lives, that points the new direction."
Richard Rohr[44]

"Mom, why are these hamburgers red? Is something wrong with them?"
"No, they are fine. They're fully cooked."
"Ugh, I hate wheat buns. Why can't we get regular ones?"
"Those are regular. They aren't wheat."
"Oh. They looked like wheat."
"Why do you keep making hamburgers if we don't have all the things we need for them? Didn't you just go to the store? We don't have lettuce again."
"Yes we do. It's right there."

---

44   Ann Belford Ulanov, "Where to Put the Bad? Where to Put the Feminine?," in *The Living God and Our Living Psyche: What Christians Can Learn from Carl Jung,* Ann Belford Ulanov and Alvin Dueck (Grand Rapids, MI: William B. Eerdmans, 2008), 55, 56.

By this point, my 16-year-old daughter had pushed me to my limit. I should have typed that last sentence in capital letters because I was not replying calmly. I had had enough of the complaints and criticism that were being dished out. I finally called her out on it and said, "Enough! Stop complaining. It's rude!"

This spiraled into a familiar dance—her feeling like I was pointing out her flaws and me feeling attacked for expressing something I wasn't okay with. I felt frustrated, watching the focus shift back onto me as if I were the one in the wrong. She stomped out, plate in hand, making a beeline to her room, but I interrupted it with "Uh-uh. You're not gonna storm away mad because I called you out on something. I'm tired of tippy toeing around you so you don't feel criticized."

It ended with me taking away her hamburger and making her sit there until she could find something nice to say. Of course, I didn't say that–I know better than to use that cheesy old line that kids hate: *"If you don't have something nice to say, don't say anything at all."* I said something more like an apology was in order, to which she replied, "I can say what you want, but I won't mean it, so why would you want me to do that?" Good point.

I walked outside for a minute and noticed my body was actually calm; there wasn't a hint of anger or hurt brewing inside of me. That was a win! I came back in, got my own plate, and went back outside to eat with my husband while she sat in the living room. As I reflected on the conversation from this neutral, uncharged place, I thought about what went well and what I could tweak. I asked my husband, "Did it sound like I was shaming her? Did I call her rude?" He replied, "I thought it went fine. My win was staying out of it."

I gave us both a bit more space and tried to get on her map—to see where she was coming from. I knew I wanted to sit down and have another conversation to repair the disconnect, coming at the conversation in a way that didn't trigger our defenses. I realized that though I hadn't directly shamed her, I was judging her. It was no wonder she didn't receive my corrections very well.

An hour later, after we'd connected around an unrelated topic and she was sitting relaxed at the dining room table, I joined her, showed interest in what she was doing, and said, "Hey, I'd love to try again and have a conversation around what happened earlier." This time, I made sure to get curious and ask questions to show her I wanted to learn and that I understood my words hadn't landed in a way that felt good to her. We ended up having a great conversation where she shared that it hurt because she'd been really working on this. She knew she could get into a negativity spiral and complain sometimes, but it felt hard to hear it pointed out—as if she always had a bad attitude. She also didn't appreciate me bringing up a situation she'd shared about a friend of hers that had gotten mad at her, telling her she complained all the time. She shared, "We all do that. I'm not the only one. Bringing up what I shared in confidence makes me not want to trust you with those things in the future."

Ouch. Received. That makes sense. Thanks for telling me that.

This was a great place to land as I realized we both felt the same thing. In the same way I wanted her to notice what was good instead of just pointing out what was wrong, she wanted exactly that, too. We all just want to be seen for who we are at our core.

We talked about confirmation bias, how our brains are wired to see the negative, and how we all have to make a conscious effort to look for and acknowledge the good in others and ourselves. We shared some examples of healthy relational dynamics where we didn't mind someone giving us constructive criticism. It was inside a supportive, secure relationship in a context where we knew the other person loved and cared for us, desiring our best. As she shared the difference between two dance teachers, I checked in to get her perspective and asked, "Do you not feel supported and encouraged by me for the most part?" She replied, "*I do.*"

We discussed what she'd like to be different the next time this came up and what would have allowed her to receive the correction. I shared what I would have liked, too. Later that night, she asked me if I wanted her to paint my nails and go watch a dance recital with her that Friday night.

Maybe you're thinking *You must have a great relationship with your teenage daughter. Mine would never do that.* Well, let's just say this has been a long road, and we've had a lot of bumps on the way. I was just as surprised by that invitation as anyone. I share all this to show the power of doing our own inner work. When we learn to distinguish our false selves from our true identities and bring to light the parts of ourselves that we judge and repress, we develop greater compassion. This process also helps us see others from a more accepting and grace-filled perspective. Healing our relationship with ourselves comes before deepening our relationships with others. It helps us learn to slow down and create space to ground ourselves in love so we can connect, offer wisdom and perspective, and activate mutual growth and respect. Our relationships, especially the closest ones, are always an opportunity for our own expansion and evolution.

No Bad Parts

"Taz is bad," my client announced, pointing to the invisible part of her sitting to her left. We were having a little fun and role playing the "parts" of herself that were in conflict in order to help her find alignment in her actions and behaviors. She had been trying to assert boundaries in a toxic relationship, but her empathetic and helpful part, which she named "Rosie," was feeling bad and sent a message to make sure this person that had been disrespecting her needs and desires felt happy and knew she cared. It turned into another one-sided phone conversation where her needs felt disregarded again.

"Taz" was the name she'd given to the part of her that was really tired of this. It was exhausted, frustrated, and pulling away, longing for space. It was the part who'd written a letter to her friend expressing her desires clearly, telling her this needed to end and asking that her wishes be respected. "Taz" was short for "Tasmanian devil," which is exactly the way she was viewing this part of herself. It was the part that could get mad, had cut people out in the past, and was able to assert itself in her job.

After having her scoot back and forth and give a voice to both parts so we could understand their motivations and allow them to learn and teach things to each other, something broke in her, and tears slipped from her eyes. "Taz is the only one who has ever protected and shown respect for me. I never realized that."

Self-judgment was transformed into self-compassion, creating space for integration, wholeness, and healing to start taking place.

We've been taught to vilify these "good" and "bad" parts, often referred to as the "ego," blaming them for tempting us or causing us to behave rashly. What if instead of judging the parts of ourselves we do not like, we followed the model of Jesus and leaned down with curiosity to get to know them and truly see them? What if we took the time to invite them to sit down and share a meal with us and listened to their story? I think we might all shed a few tears when we come to realize they arose as our protectors in the moments of our deepest pain.

A healthy ego and these parts that serve to keep us alive are a part of God's design. Without them, none of us would be around today. Yes, their energy can get aggressive, domineering, controlling, manipulating, or self-abasing, but underneath their "sinful" behavior lies the desire to guard our vulnerability.

What We Resist Persists

Jeannie, a client who was part of a Group Coaching program I co-led, shared the shifts she was experiencing as she began changing the way she was viewing and relating to herself and her emotions: "I've always resisted and pushed away my negative emotions, viewing them as bad and something to fix. I'm just now starting to realize that that only makes them grow stronger. I'm learning that when I witness them and give a voice to them, everything softens, and my whole body relaxes."

Compassion and love have a way of doing that. Just as "fighting" and trying to prove ourselves triggers people's defenses and escalates arguments, trying to "fight" our "demons," our cancers, and our own flesh as if it's evil and something to cast out only serves to strengthen the energy of these protective parts. Going to war against our own bodies and souls never leads to peace within. It just amplifies anxiety and turns on inflammation. No wonder so many women struggle with autoimmune diseases. Our bodies are receiving the message that our very flesh is something to be attacked.

In his book No Bad Parts, author Richard Schwartz, PhD, recounts an experience that fundamentally changed his perspective on people.[45] This transformative insight contributed to the development of Internal Family Systems (IFS) theory, a model that has been reshaping the field of psychology for decades and played a significant role in my Mastery Coaching Training. He experienced a breakthrough one day with a woman that was engaging in self-harm. In his exasperation, he let go of trying to control her actions and shifted into curiosity and compassion toward the part of her responsible for the cutting. In that judgment-free zone, it opened up and shared it was only trying to control her rage so she wouldn't get abused more. As he

---

45 Schwartz, Richard C. *No Bad Parts: Healing Trauma and Restoring Wholeness with the Internal Family Systems Model*. Sounds True, 2021.

reflected his appreciation, she broke into tears, finally being seen as the hero instead of judged and labeled as a demonic force.

Dr. Swartz shares why this approach is so effective: "Through a Christian lens, through Internal Family Systems, people wind up doing to the inner world what Jesus did in the outer–they go to inner exiles and enemies with love, heal them, and bring them home, just as he did with the lepers, the poor and the outcasts." He encourages us to see these parts for what they are: spiritual beings that deserve to be treated as sacred parts of the soul. This is so important if we truly want to be a light in a world full of hurting people–a bridge for human souls instead of a force that perpetuates division and judgment.

"How we relate in the inner world will be how we relate in the outer. If we can appreciate and have compassion for our parts, even the ones we've considered to be enemies, we can do the same for people who resemble them. On the other hand, if we hate or disdain our parts, we'll do the same with anyone who reminds us of them."

Getting to Know Our Shadow Self

We all come into the world open and free of judgment, but as we get older, we have experiences that cause us to start judging ourselves. We receive messages about what's acceptable and what's not, and those unacceptable things about ourselves are pushed into the shadows. "The Shadow Self" represents the darker, hidden aspects of our personality that we may not be consciously aware of. According to Carl Jung, the Shadow Self is not inherently negative or evil; rather, it is a natural part of the human psyche that serves a purpose.[46] The Shadow can act as a reservoir of untapped potential and creativity, as well as a source of wisdom and insight into our deepest selves. However, when

---

46 Bastos, Filipe. "Shadow Self: How Knowing Your Dark Side Can Help You in Life." *MindOwl*, 1 Nov. 2019, https://mindowl.org/shadow-self/.

neglected or denied, the Shadow can manifest in destructive ways, such as through mental health issues, addictive behaviors, or interpersonal conflicts: [47] "It's what our ego deems as negative, and relationally risky. And it often is, but it often holds repressed traits that may have been invalidated or minimized by others; beautiful parts, inspired dreams, hopes and creativity that we have left to languish."

One of the best things we can do is work toward accepting and integrating the shadow rather than continually rejecting it. When we learn to bring our shadows back into the light, we regain potential energy that has been held and contained. Instead of constant internal tug of wars, we enjoy greater peace and confidence. Instead of being unconsciously driven by the feelings and needs that have been pushed down into the shadows, we find the courage to move forward as conscious co-creators of our lives. The Shadow Self holds the parts of yourself that are difficult to accept: the parts seen as bad.

Seeing Your Shadow in Others

My daughter is my Shadow Self. She embodies all the parts of me that I never allowed in myself and have been working on resurrecting and integrating. These things include assertiveness and being able to ask for what I need, receiving things without feeling guilty or like I need to give something in return, putting boundaries around my empathy, and saying no without feeling selfish. That also makes my daughter one of my greatest triggers and forces me to confront my own unhealed wounds. In my efforts to never be perceived as rude or uncaring, I shoved my assertiveness and strength into the basement of my soul, labeled it the enemy, and judged anyone that reflected it back at me. That

---

47 Bastos, "Shadow Self."

works pretty good until you find yourself judging your own child and freaking out, thinking, *Did I raise a narcissist?*

For the record, I do not think my daughter is a narcissist. When she is grounded and secure in her own self-love, she is my hero and role model. (Whoa. Just typing that brought tears to my eyes.) God often gives us a glimpse of what He sees from on high when we least expect it. That flood of emotion is like a releasing of the scales on my eyes.

Maybe you're getting caught up on that whole "self love" thing and thinking, *Wait a minute. You can't say that. Self-love is selfish and prideful.* I almost went back and changed it to "true self" so you wouldn't get hung up on it, but I'm leaving it. That's my healing work—learning to stop seeing loving ourselves as wrong, as something to be erased and covered over with false humility or self-negation.

It reminds me of when I first met my husband. He, too, reflected parts of my Shadow Self. I was drawn to his confidence, yet I couldn't help but make it my mission to pull him down from the clouds and "humble" him. You know, shrink him to a size I thought was more appropriate—less cocky and more humble, like me!

Our souls are always seeking opportunities to create the circumstances we need to practice healing and growth. This is why we are often drawn to people who reflect our unhealed wounds and unmet needs, like iron clippings to a magnet. These relationships can act as mirrors, showing us the parts of ourselves that we have hidden away or judged harshly. This dynamic is not just about romantic relationships but also extends to our children and friendships.

This attraction can be good and bad. It either leads us into toxic dynamics where we're butting heads and reenacting our trauma over and over again or opportunities for both parties to learn and grow through their interactions. This unconscious reenactment, also known as trauma bonding, replicates the conditions of our original wounds. We do this in an attempt to resolve and heal our old pains.

Through understanding these concepts, I'm now able to separate my "trigger" and defensive reactions as I realize the familiarity of them. Those stings of rejection are more about the past than the present, and they are a trailhead to my transformation. When my daughter says or does something that I would never do, such as replying "no, thanks" when I ask if she wants to help me prepare the Thanksgiving meal or watch a Christmas movie together, I focus on her apparent lack of consideration for my desire to share these experiences. In such moments, I recognize it as an opportunity to update the outdated strategies I'm using to connect with her and reevaluate the stories that arise from my hurt feelings. Stories like, *How rude. How selfish. Where is her empathy and compassion? Her sense of care and helpfulness? Why doesn't she want to spend time with me? She must really not like me to never want to be with me,"* or *"I really screwed up somewhere as a parent for her to not have more regard for others."*

My mind goes backward into the past, loading up on nostalgia, searching for memories of when things were better: *I miss my other daughter. She would have watched Little Women with me. She would have helped me make the pies. I miss my sisters. I wish they were here.* Loneliness settles in my home like an unwanted guest during the holidays.

The problem with this is my brain and nervous system are always doing the very thing my daughter and I discussed: using bias, filtering, and finding evidence to confirm the stories and beliefs my body is holding. When our core wound and greatest fear is rejection, we will see someone's choice to put up boundaries and say no as a validation of our unlovability. This perceived abandonment triggers our deepest fears of being unwanted, flawed, and repulsive. My daughter embodies qualities I suppressed in myself, forcing me to confront and integrate those parts. Similarly, my husband's confidence attracted me because it was something I needed to further develop. Understanding this can be a powerful tool for personal growth. Instead of seeing these relationships as mere sources of pain or conflict, we can view them as opportunities for healing. By recognizing and working through our reactions, we can transform our triggers into paths toward wholeness and self-love. This is the essence of getting to know our Shadow Self: seeing our relationships as catalysts for the healing journey our souls are on.

Seek Supportive Relationships for Healthy Integration

It's crucial to discern the difference between relationships that are supportive and opportunities for healing, growth, and corrective experiences and toxic ones that perpetuate harm, unhealthy patterns, and abuse.

Here are some guidelines to help discern the difference:

1. **Safety and Respect:** A relationship that fosters healing is based on mutual respect and safety. If a relationship involves consistent disrespect, fear, or harm, it's not conducive to healing and likely perpetuates trauma.
2. **Growth and Empowerment:** Healing relationships encourage personal growth and empowerment. They support you in becoming more of who you truly are. In contrast, toxic relationships often involve control, manipulation, and diminishing your sense of self-worth.
3. **Boundaries:** In healthy relationships, boundaries are respected and valued. You feel comfortable setting and maintaining boundaries. Toxic relationships, on the other hand, often involve boundary violations and pressure to compromise your values or well-being.

4. **Emotional Regulation:** A relationship that aids healing helps you regulate your emotions and deal with triggers constructively. Unhealthy relationships frequently leave you feeling more anxious, depressed, or emotionally unstable.

By being mindful of these differences, you can better navigate your relationships with discernment while prioritizing your safety, well-being, and self-respect.

GOOD GIRL RX: Get to Know and Integrate Your Shadow Self

Embracing the parts of ourselves we've hidden—the shadow we've labeled as "bad" or "wrong"—isn't just about feeling whole; it's a profound step toward real healing. Each part, even those we've judged, holds a piece of our story and a drive to protect us. By learning to see these parts with compassion instead of criticism, we create room to breathe, reducing the constant tension and internal stress that comes from battling ourselves. This matters deeply in our journey to heal, not just mentally but physically. When we stop the inner fight, our bodies start to let go of the stress they've been carrying. Our nervous systems can rest. Instead of resisting ourselves, we begin to feel more at peace, creating an openness that lets us show up for others from a place of true connection and grace. As you move forward, remember: healing is not about fixing what's "broken." It's about finally honoring the whole person you've always been.

Reflection Questions:

1. Think of a part of yourself you've judged or tried to hide. What if that part was trying to protect you in some way? What might change if you approached it with curiosity and compassion instead of criticism?
2. Think about a time when you felt frustrated or annoyed with yourself, like when you didn't speak up, set a boundary, or lost your temper with your child. Imagine if this were another mother in the same situation. What might be some really good reasons she held back or lost her cool? How might you see her with understanding and compassion rather than judgment? What would you have to let go of to look at yourself in the same way?
3. Think of someone who recently triggered a reaction in you. What if instead of focusing on their behavior, you looked at the heart beneath it? How might that help you respond differently with more peace and understanding?

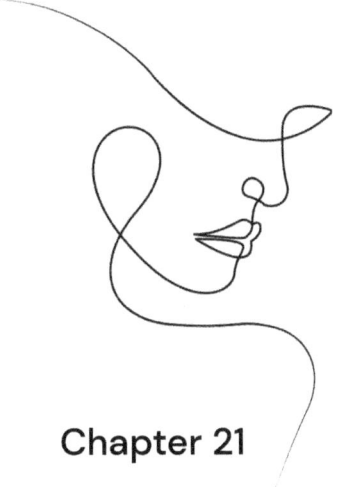

Chapter 21

Breaking the Rules: No More Supposed To's

"...that they should seek God, and perhaps feel their way toward him and find him. Yet he is actually not far from each one of us..."
Acts 17:27, ESV

Something broke in me this morning, and I had to grab a paper towel to blot my eyes and blow my nose. I was reading a devotional from Bob Goff's book, *Live in Grace, Walk in Love*,[48] and felt this beautiful permission slip handed to me that said, *Just sit, listen, and see people; see to the heart of the matter. That's it; nothing more.* My whole body slipped into agreement, and a weight was lifted off of me that I didn't even know was there.

I'd grabbed the book and brought it to the kitchen table that morning, hoping to find words of life that could untangle the confusion clouding my heart and mind but not really expecting it to. I just knew the simple rhythm of reading and reflecting as

---

48 Goff, Bob. *Live in Grace, Walk in Love: A 365-Day Journey*. Thomas Nelson, 2019.

I held a warm cup of coffee was something I could be certain would ground me in the midst of the unknowns floating around in my head.

I had no idea why the words moved me so deeply, but as I continued reading, it became clear. All I ever wanted was to love people, sit, listen, witness, and provide a judgment-free zone to help them get to the heart of what was troubling them. Why couldn't it be that simple? Why did I always have to complicate it?

As I reflected on that question, a new emotion arose with a surge of thoughts insisting to be heard: *I'm so freaking tired of trying to figure out what I am supposed to be doing and who I'm supposed to be serving and the problem I am supposed to be solving. I am so done with the 'supposed to's!*

Rage escaped from my chest, erupting in bursts like steam when the valve on the instant pot is set to release. Those stupid supposed to's had taken up so much of my time, my life, and my sanity. I just want to love people in *this* way. But here I was again, questioning, doubting, second-guessing the direction I was so confident of just a few days before; a too common pattern for me. I call it my habit of forgetfulness: a habit I can't seem to shake no matter how many vision boards I make.

The devotional continued with the example of Jesus breaking all the rules with the woman at the well, and I thought, *Yes! That is what I want too! I am done following all the rules*—the 'business' rules, the 'church' rules, the 'how to be a good mom, successful entrepreneur, and writer rules. Rules just drive me deeper into my head, where I get stuck trying to make sure I'm using my time and energy in a way that's helpful and good; I lose not only my confidence but attunement with my internal GPS.

All those stupid rules do is reinforce my mind's relentless search for validation, and that search is never productive. It's like searching for the keys you misplaced and have already spent over an hour lifting every cushion, digging in every pocket, and moving the car seat forward and backward while you strain to feel for them in the crevices your eyes can't see. That same frustration of knowing they have to be somewhere, the irritation about how much time is passing, feeling like you're going crazy, wanting to just give up, but not being able to relax or do anything else because you know you're stuck. I do not want to search for the fricken keys anymore!

Yes, I really wanted to say something else right there, but those stupid rules made me edit it. And here's what else starts arising even with that strong intuitive gut declaration. I hear, *Seek and ye shall find. Knock and the door shall be opened,* and that word "seek" starts twisting itself around my body's desire to stop the relentless pursuit.

I read a comment in another Christian book recently that felt like an oxymoron. The author spoke of laying down our striving and inviting God's strength to be imparted to us, and the suggested pathway to that was through passionate pursuit of Him. I guess it depends on the way you read and interpret the word "pursuit" and what that leads you to do, but I see too many "Good Girls" pursuing and loving God with the same seeking behaviors they learned as young children: behaviors that were developed to ensure relational safety and security. While those are necessary and effective to get a young child's needs met, as adults, they block the freedom of confident exploration and growing in self-trust.

I have to continually remind myself that I can call off the search! I don't need to pursue God. He is within me! His presence, peace, and inspiration are not something I have to seek, but, rather, can lean into. I find it when I remind myself that I can surrender that outdated strategy! I'm learning to replace the pursuit with presence and my attempts to love Him with the invitation to let Him love me.

It's often so unconscious that I don't even realize I'm getting caught up in it again. I've come a long way in learning to shift out of this pattern of seeking external validation for my directions, choices, and actions, but it has a way of grabbing me by the ankle and shackling me, no matter how hard I try to shake it loose. Sometimes, I get so angry at the church, society, and the Scriptures that have been programmed into me, playing like a broken record, hindering me from embodying the confidence I need to actually lean into love and find that validation within me.

Seeking Validation

I used to scan my Bible, flipping pages, searching for direction until I realized God didn't work that way. I thought "seeking" meant seeking Scripture, so I would dig and come away disappointed if my question or specific life challenge wasn't addressed. I was desperately looking for validation for what God wanted me to do. It wasn't until a few years into married life that I learned to seek Him in a way that led to peace. What if the seeking looks more like tuning in through solitude, rest, and presence instead of the analytical search our minds get caught in an effort to feel safe?

When we're young, we often become sensitive to our environments, reading the cues around us and using that feedback to direct our actions. This hypervigilance, scanning, and reading people is a really important survival response, but if we want to enjoy the freedom Christ died to give us access to, we have to update those neural pathways that were wired in as kids.

The first step to breaking free from the rules, supposed to's, and constant seeking is to let the part of you that learned to do this to feel relationally secure know that this habit is no longer serving the purpose it was designed for. If you ever feel like your life is a constant search for direction, validation, clarity, or confirmation, you get this. It sucks, doesn't it? Why can't we just live and move and be without needing to know what the crap we are "supposed" to be doing?

This problem is one of the greatest sources of anxiety and chronic physical symptoms in women. What if we all just gave ourselves permission to *call off the search*? To stop striving so hard to figure out what we're supposed to be doing and simply allow ourselves to *be*? This isn't about abandoning the part of us that seeks clarity; it's about recognizing the underlying need: to feel safe in the midst of uncertainty. The next time you find yourself 'seeking direction,' use that as an invitation to pause and check in with your body. Is the energy one of curiosity and exploration or frantic searching? Stop and notice what your mind is doing in response to that, and approach yourself with curiosity and self-compassion like you would if you found a lost child in the shopping mall. This shift takes practice and patience, but it opens the door to the freedom and peace we all long for. God isn't asking us to play this exhausting game of hide and seek. He's already here, within us, inviting us to lean into His presence where true security is found—a presence we access not through our heads but by grounding in our bodies, where the Spirit dwells.

The Freedom To Be Where We Are

Last week, I had a chance to step away from all of the questioning and spend a week taking care of my granddaughter while her parents were at a conference. We got to play, go on adventures, cuddle with books, and explore the city together. It felt so right, so sweet, so easy, and nice. What might open up if we could all find the freedom to lean into the rhythms of life and be with each other? What if we had the time to sit, listen, and really see each other? To be together without an agenda, without the pressure to please, perform, or perfect anything? Nothing pulling at us or tearing our insides apart? It's the thing we all want more of—well, at least it is for me—and I know it's the message God is whispering as He beckons us into this sweet I AM where that clarity, direction, and validation we've been seeking is found without lifting a finger. It just arises like the dew on the grass, like the keys that just show up the next day when we stop looking for them.

Kacy's Story: Learning to Sit in the Tension

Kacy was a young girl who came with us on a mission trip my husband led. She had been diagnosed with Celiac Disease and had been reading some books on the stress-disease connection and autoimmunity, allowing for some great conversations around our mutual passion. During a long layover at the airport on the way home, she shared her perspective on how "Good Girl" conditioning impacted her and what she was working on to heal: "I never break the rules. I mean, it's good to be a 'Good Girl.' It's peaceful. If you don't break any rules, you won't be in a position to get in trouble." Placing her hand on her chest, she continued, "When I was three, I knocked a plant into the sink and vividly remember that feeling of, 'Oh my gosh. I made a mess, and I can't clean it up.' My dad saw it later and asked who did it and I lied and blamed it on the cat. I got spanked for that. Disappointing my dad like that made my heart sink. I never wanted to get in trouble again. My sister was the opposite. She got a B once, and my dad told her she could do better. She worked so hard but felt like a failure and eventually stopped trying, feeling like she could never be good enough."

"When I first started my job, it was hard to say no. I worked ten-hour days and always said yes, even if I knew it was a waste of time and energy. I never got a 'thanks for doing that.' I know I shouldn't rely on them to tell me 'good job,' but a few words of affirmation would be nice after all the work I put in. I've grown in this area and am in a place of power where I can say no now. My first thought is still, 'He's not going to like me. I won't be seen as a team player,' but I'm setting that boundary anyway. I don't work late anymore."

"I had the same problem with my dad but finally realized he wouldn't do the same for me; there was no reciprocity. I've gotten stronger, and he doesn't like it, but I'm learning to sit in the tension of him not being okay with what I say or do. I still question myself, wondering, *'Am I doing the right thing?'*"

Kacy was working on what all "Good Girls" need to learn to do: sit in the tension of others not being okay with us. That's challenging when your peace and attachment security has been hinged on whether people are pleased with you. It can feel like you're going to get in trouble, and just like Kacy, that doesn't just make our hearts sink; it can feel so threatening we lie to protect ourselves from it.

Children don't lie to be 'bad'; they lie to avoid the shame and separation anxiety that comes from sensing our disappointment. They need the safety to be honest and the freedom to say, 'Oops, sorry!'—and to correct themselves without fear of our reaction.

Julie's Story: Rules and More Rules

Julie's story offers another layer of insight into how rigid rules and high expectations can shape a person's life, often with lasting consequences. Like Kacy, Julie wrestled with the weight of Good Girl conditioning, but her journey took her through an entirely different landscape of challenges.

"Growing up as a preacher's kid, I was immersed in a world of strict rules and high expectations. Shorts, makeup, and jewelry were all off-limits. Even playing softball was deemed too enticing for a good girl like me. The pressure to be perfect was relentless; after all, only the perfect could hope to enter heaven. So, I became the perfect teen, never daring to drink or step out of line. But perfection came at a cost. My parents, also raised in this rigid environment, instilled in me the belief that being perfect was the only way to be accepted. Naive and gullible, I had not experienced enough of the real world to see through people's facades, leaving me vulnerable to hurt."

My upbringing instilled a strong sense of right and wrong, rooted in the best intentions of my parents. They raised me with values they believed would protect and guide me, but those well-meaning rules and expectations unintentionally created mental roadblocks. These roadblocks shaped how I viewed myself and others, often leading me to judge anyone who didn't meet the high standards of perfection I felt were necessary.

When my own children began making choices that didn't align with the rules I had enforced, I struggled to let go of control. I feared what would happen if they strayed too far from the path I had set for them. Despite my efforts to protect them, I couldn't shield them—or myself—from pain.

I married someone who seemed safe, only to discover he was anything but. He was abusive, both physically and emotionally, and even harmed my daughter in ways I never could have imagined. I was blindsided by his transformation from someone who appeared to be a good man into a manipulative monster. After the divorce, I found myself grappling with deep guilt and self-blame. I kept asking myself, 'How could I have missed the signs? Why didn't I protect my children better?' But the truth is, I was naive, too trusting, and ill-equipped to see the truth until it was too late.

Now, as I work to navigate the fallout of my past, I find myself estranged from my adult children. They don't understand the pain I endured or the mistakes I made trying to be a good mother. I long for their love and acceptance but fear I may never receive it."

"My journey to healing has been fraught with challenges. Chronic stress, digestive issues, and emotional eating are just a few of the physical manifestations of my pain. Sleep disturbances and panic attacks further compound my struggles, often leaving me feeling overwhelmed and isolated. I've come a long way.

Ten years ago, I would have worn out a highlighter on the good girl syndrome quiz. I've learned to say no. I still deal with these things, but it's not as bad. I still worry about upsetting others and lose sleep trying to figure out what I did wrong. I still deal with low self-worth, comparing myself to people that are younger, skinnier, and don't have wrinkles and gray hair. I'm harder on myself than anyone else and can be really self-critical. Fear of abandonment is still huge and very difficult. I'm afraid of being all alone if something happens to my husband. Internalized self-blame is not as bad, but it's still there, especially regarding my kids. Some things are better, but it's still there. I don't care as much about what people think–you either like me or you don't. I think it's shifted because my circumstances have shifted. I have an easier job and a better husband now. Despite the darkness that has overshadowed much of my life, I hold onto hope. Healing is possible, even if it feels out of reach at times."

Julie's story reminds us that healing doesn't happen overnight, nor does it mean everything will suddenly be perfect. It's a journey of learning to live with the tension of what was, what is, and what we hope for. For those walking through similar challenges, it's a reminder that progress, no matter how small, is still progress. Each step toward reclaiming your voice, setting boundaries, or finding moments of joy is a victory worth celebrating.

Her story also speaks to the importance of breaking free from the rules and expectations that have weighed us down. That's something I experienced firsthand in a moment that, though small, felt monumental to me at the time—a tiny act of rebellion that I'll never forget.

A Taste of Rebellion

I thought I was going to die the day my friends finally convinced me to sneak off campus for lunch my Senior year. They were like, "Kate, we do it all the time and never get caught. It's no big deal. We're just going to go pick it up, and we will be back before anyone even knows we're even gone." That did nothing to soothe my conscience. Dread churned in my stomach as I huddled on the floorboard of my friend's red convertible, convinced that every passing vehicle would somehow expose my act of rebellion. When we finally got to McDonald's, I let out an exhale and laughed out loud as I climbed out and let myself be seen again. I was nervous the whole time and anxious to get back before my absence was detected, but it was so worth the freedom I tasted as I munched on those greasy fries and sipped my chocolate shake.

Breaking the rules isn't just about defiance or bending boundaries—it's about overcoming fear and reclaiming our freedom to act autonomously. Breaking the rules, even in small ways, can be essential for maintaining balance and preserving our mental well-being. While rules often serve as guidelines for societal order and personal discipline, rigid adherence to them can lead to feelings of restriction and dissatisfaction. Allowing ourselves the freedom to break a few rules now and then serves as a reminder that we are human, imperfect beings capable of making our own choices and finding joy in spontaneity. By embracing these small acts of rebellion, we reclaim a sense of autonomy over our lives, fostering creativity, resilience, and self-expression. Moreover, breaking the rules in harmless ways can serve as a form of self-care, providing much-needed relief from the pressures of conformity and perfectionism. So, whether it's indulging in a guilty pleasure or simply marching to the beat of our own drum, a little rebellion now and then can be just what the doctor ordered for our mental and emotional well-being.

Here are some ideas to get you jump-started!

- Take a day off from your usual exercise routine and spend it lounging in bed or exploring nature at your leisure.
- Play a practical joke on someone.

- Sneak food into the movie theater.
- Let yourself cuss when you're alone and let all your feelings out.
- Skip church, a meeting, or something else you don't usually let yourself miss and indulge in a day of spontaneity or do nothing!
- Call in sick to work and take a mental health day.
- Leave the dishes in the sink overnight.
- Stay up late binge-watching your favorite shows or reading a good book.
- When you have to take the boring annual compliance test at work that you've taken umpteenth times, skip the reading and just keep taking the quiz until you finally get a passing score.

Listen to what these "Good Girls" shared about breaking the rules to inspire you more!

"Taking a nap in the middle of the day! That would set my mother on fire if she caught you sleeping when you could be doing something productive."

"I bought myself a red Mustang convertible!"

"Giving myself permission to say 'no' has always been a tough one for me. I never want to be seen as uncaring, selfish, or self-centered and have often taken on way more than I should have to keep from disappointing others."

"I was staying with my very proper aunt over the summer and found a Harlequin romance hidden in her bedroom. She was reading it! I was shocked! While she was at work, I would sneak it out and read it. It was a guilty thrill at 15. To this day, a good romance is my go-to if I need to escape."

"I stayed up late reading books, mostly romance novels. It was my escape. I wasn't allowed to have many friends, and my parents were so strict about who could visit, even if they were from church. My aunt thought that was crazy and secretly invited my friend for a sleepover without my parents knowing. When my stepdad came over unexpectedly, my friend hid under the bed. My heart was pounding, but we laughed so hard after he left. She was my partner in crime, and I miss her dearly."

GOOD GIRL RX: Reconnect to Your Internal Compass

Sometimes, when we're caught in the endless 'supposed to's' and the need to get everything just right, we lose touch with the Spirit's wisdom that's already inside us. That voice of love never pushes or pulls us into stress or self-doubt. It's a gentle presence, inviting us back into connection. The first step is to notice when you're seeking from your head and use that as a cue to pause and get grounded in the body where you can access the leadership of the Spirit. You'll know it when you're there, as you'll find curiosity, clarity, creativity, confidence- all the lovely fruits of the Spirit that feel so much better than overthinking and anxiety!

Reflection Questions:

1. Have you ever felt trapped by the expectations of what you think you *should* be doing? What would happen if you gave yourself permission to let go of those "supposed to's" and gave yourself more freedom?
2. Think of a time when you were searching for answers or direction. What would change if you stopped seeking external validation and trusted that you already have access to what you need inside of you? Where do you feel resistance to this? What thoughts arise?
3. Is there a small "rule" you could break this week to remind yourself of your freedom? How could this act of rebellion help you reconnect with your true self?

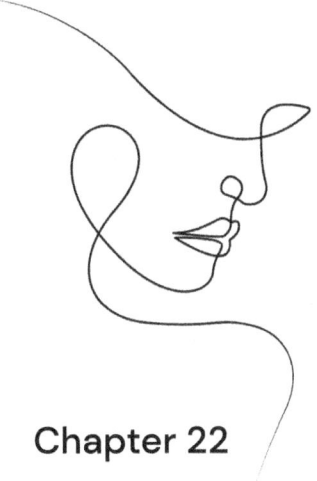

Chapter 22

Stepping Into Empowerment: Moving Beyond Good Girl Syndrome

"Don't ask yourself what the world needs. Ask yourself what makes you come alive, and go do that, because what the world needs is people who have come alive."
Howard Thurman[49]

Riley had been serving overseas in India for eight months when Covid hit. She had to rush to the airport, catching the last flight out of the country right before they closed the borders. Since she'd gotten back to the States, she was struggling to breathe and nothing from a medical perspective seemed to be helping. When I jumped on a Zoom call with her and a mutual

---

49 Bailie, Gil. Violence Unveiled: Humanity at the Crossroads. The Crossroad Publishing Company, 1996.

friend to see if I could point her in the right direction, she shared, "I haven't been able to sleep in weeks; every time I lay down, my body is coursing with adrenaline. I have heart palpitations and pain with breathing every day. I'd like to find answers to what's going on with my breathing, get relief, and learn better coping skills for living healthy in light of what my body has been doing. I haven't found anything that's truly alleviated the anxiety and adrenaline, nor the pain."

She'd been trying to walk, process her thoughts with friends, yoga, taking melatonin, having a glass of wine before bed, and using the inhaler that had been prescribed to her. She was also going to counseling and taking medication for anxiety and depression. "I just want to sleep through the night, run again, and get back to full-time ministry without worrying about having a panic attack and not being able to get enough air in." Nighttime was a trigger for her, and when she laid down for bed, she became flooded with anxiety.

Within thirty minutes of listening to the backstory and what had been going on in the preceding weeks and months, it became clear a danger alarm had been going off in her body in the midst of all the uncertainty. Since she'd gotten home, she'd been feeling really unsettled: "I don't have a permanent place to call home, have a very loosely defined job, and am having to depend financially on other people giving money to me."

Can you feel all of that with her?

She had a history of anxiety. She pushed herself to overcome it and go live overseas. She had been struggling with her life's direction, and saying yes to serving in India helped her feel more settled, as she believed it was something God would approve of. Although she was enjoying the work and feeling good about having a purpose, she'd struggled with feeling safe and had a hard time opening up to anyone on her team about her fears. Her body had already been expressing what she couldn't through an irregular cycle the weeks before she got on that plane and was now shouting even louder.

From Self-Doubt to Freedom and Confidence

Gaining an understanding about what was happening in her body got her out of uncertainty, restoring a much-needed sense of safety. When I met with her the next week, she shared, "I slept like a baby that night and have been sleeping well since then."

She also realized the steroid inhaler had been making it worse, amplifying the adrenaline that was already coursing through her body. She weaned back off of that and began doing things like nature walks, coffee dates, and other mindfulness practices to bring more cues of safety to her body and settle into a parasympathetic state. Over the next several sessions, we began uncovering the root of her anxiety and why that experience had been so unsettling for her. Her decision to serve in India had been a safe one. When that certainty was stripped away with no time to even be in choice about it, she lost her anchor and compass. Her need to *"do the right thing and what God wanted"* was tied to her sense of security. I understand that need personally and see it in so many women. We're always asking the question, *Am I doing the right thing? Am I in God's will?*

One session, we traced the body sensations she experienced around that question and found a young memory when she was feeling the same way. She was lying on the couch, lost in a good book, when an uncle standing over her questioned how she was spending her time. She immediately put the book up, feeling like what she was doing was not approved of. As we continued the timeline exercise, she found more memories where she'd been self-conscious about her choices and was able to connect the dots to her present challenge around making decisions and trusting herself. She shared how this same thing had been affecting her dating relationships and how she'd been praying for a man who would help her make good choices and stay in God's will. She didn't feel like she could trust herself and wanted someone who would make sure she didn't go astray. She'd never gotten past a first date as her analytical mind sat across the table like a protective parent, assessing them to make sure they were good for her.

As we worked through that, she began letting go and started allowing herself more freedom to enjoy their company without all that pressure to *"get it right."* Letting go of that pressure allowed her to say yes to a date while we were working together, and that yes led to a really big yes when that guy she opened up to got down on one knee and proposed to her a year later.

Her new confidence gave her the freedom to say many more yes's, like staying in the States, taking a job with her degree in social work, getting in touch with her creative side, exploring her passions for art, and starting her own business. Every time I see one of her Instagram posts sharing her art, I smile and see the image of the little girl in overalls and pigtails that had raised her hand in a "parts" meeting exercise to share her creative ideas when she was feeling fearful of a decision. Her words say it all: "I've learned how to explore my options with open hands. It's okay to head one way, explore, and go a different direction. I can try, fail, and try again. That makes me smile and even giggle."

Discovering and aligning with our purpose can often feel like a game of hide and seek, where the person we're searching for is not even participating—they're off reading a book while we continue to look under every pillow and behind every door. It's like, *Hey God, I'm willing to do whatever, but I kind of need you to show me. How the heck am I supposed to figure it out if you don't tell me already?*

Here's the thing: our purposes are not hiding, and as Riley and I both learned, God is not holding His hands behind Him with our purpose in one, waiting for us to pick the right one. In the same way, God showed me that when we see things from His perspective, we can't get it wrong. As soon as we let go of the fear that we're going to choose the wrong thing, we find the freedom to choose what makes our hearts sing!

Breaking free to walk in our purpose and experience fulfillment within it always starts with restoring the security we need to lie on the couch and read a fiction book and trust that our hearts can lead us. Finding purpose is a process of exploration. It's okay if we try something and decide it's not life-giving for us. Just keep taking a step forward, explore, try it on, and give yourself permission to pivot. Sometimes fulfillment jumps out and says, *"Here I am!"* when you stop trying so hard to find it. Start letting yourself follow the lights outside your window.

No need to strain and try to figure them out, just put on a coat, start taking a walk, and let yourself dance on your way there.

GOOD GIRL RX: Restore Self-Trust

Give yourself permission to explore without the fear of getting it wrong. Trust your desires, follow what feels life-giving, and take small steps toward what excites you. If something doesn't work out, that's okay—allow yourself to pivot and try again. The freedom to choose comes from trusting yourself, not from waiting for the perfect answer.

Reflection Questions:

1. Riley realized that trusting herself was key to finding peace and confidence. What decisions in your life have you been hesitant to make because you're afraid of getting it wrong? How might trusting yourself more open up new possibilities for you?
2. Riley was caught in the cycle of trying to "get it right" with every decision. Do you ever feel like you need to make the perfect choice or be on the "right" path? How would your life change if you let go of the pressure to be perfect and embraced trying, failing, and trying again?
3. Riley discovered that fulfillment came when she stopped trying so hard to find it. What would happen if you stopped over-analyzing and simply followed the invitation right in front of you? Where might your heart lead you if you gave it the freedom to explore?

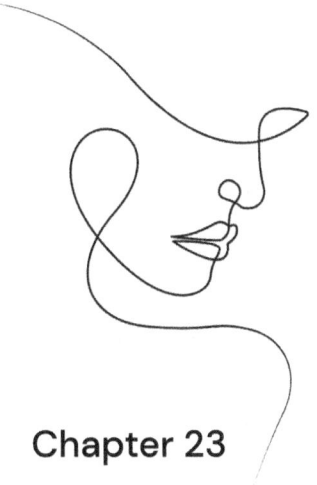

Chapter 23

The Best You: The Good Girl Whose Story Helped Another

"As we let our own light shine, we unconsciously give other people permission to do the same."
Marianne Williamson[50]

When I interviewed women for this book, one of the things I heard many times was, *"I love books, but the problem is that I get to the end and then think, okay, great, but how do I apply this to my life?"*

I hope the tools provided throughout this journey are valuable resources you can revisit and utilize. However, I also recognize that having too many tools can be overwhelming. If we're not careful, we might try to "fix" ourselves with these resources instead of trusting our intuition. It's important to allow ourselves to move

---

50 Williamson, Marianne. *A Return to Love: Reflections on the Principles of "A Course in Miracles."* HarperCollins, 1992.

forward from a place of faith and empowerment. My prayer is that the stories I've shared serve to inspire, provide hope, clarity, and greater understanding for yourself and others. Allow what you've digested to settle and be integrated. Take some walks, journal, connect with other women, and talk about your insights and discoveries.

Moving beyond "Good Girl Syndrome" is a process like untangling matted hair after a rough night of sleep; it's better to use a gentle conditioner than to force your way through it. Be gentle with yourself and trust that you are exactly where you are supposed to be.

I really wanted to be able to give you a four-step system, but I knew that would serve to do the opposite of what you needed. Healing isn't linear, and there is no magic formula you can apply or perfect prayer you can pray. It's more like peeling an onion one layer at a time, stepping into more and more trust along the way. I can't tell you what to do, as healing for the "Good Girl" is all about finding your own intuitive prescription and trusting the guidance within you.

My favorite part about being an Empowerment Coach is that I don't have to have all the answers! I simply get to guide women into the insights they already know but aren't acting on and provide the tools, support, mirroring, and accountability they need to break through the resistance. That's my prayer for you, too. That this book serves to grow your confidence in the same way mine is bolstered when I read something that reminds me I'm not alone, and someone says what I've been thinking but am too afraid to express. I pray my story and the voices of the women who courageously shared their journeys undergirds you like a parasail harness and skyrockets you to a view that inspires your next steps.

Empowerment, by its very definition, is a process of becoming stronger and more confident as you journey through life. It's a choice we make every day when we check in with ourselves and get curious about our "come from." Whether we're awaiting test results and feeling like things are out of our control and we're at the mercy of our circumstances, or we're frustrated with a family member or boss, thinking, *They'll never understand. Nothing is ever going to change. I'm stuck. This is my lot in life.* That's a pretty good sign we're in a place of disempowerment. Nothing changes when we're unplugged in that way. Moving forward is about becoming the co-creator of our lives and realizing we are not passive observers that have to wait and pray that things change. We get to join with God and step into our creative capacity to ignite change from within!

Empowerment requires us to stand in front of the mirror and realize we are no longer children who need to be led around by a leash. We don't need to wait for a cue or command. We get to lead ourselves and follow our noises!

In the process of writing this book, I've experienced the power of presence and trust in a way like never before. I let go of all the expectations to show up on social media every day, write my weekly newsletters, get my website improved, stay on the timeline my publishing company set, and I allowed myself the grace and permission to focus on doing what I already knew to do and what was right in front of me. It took me months to get here, and if you asked my husband and my body, they'd both tell you it was no easy feat to move beyond the resistance that is allowing for that today. Every day, every minute, is an intentional decision to shift back into connection where I can find the resources I need and move forward in empowerment and strength. If you were a bird in my yard, you'd see me stopping to breathe, placing a hand on my chest, feeling the wind on my face every time I start to feel rattled, annoyed, frustrated, or stuck in my head.

Moving forward is all about those little pauses and self check-in's. It's feeling the rubber band pulling us back and down, noticing it, and relaxing instead of fighting against it. When we do, we can stop and see what has a hold of us and unite with love to untangle it.

Journaling Our Way Forward

Journaling became a powerful tool for me during a season when I felt stuck, and it's still my go-to resource. It helps me see with new clarity and perspective, ignites hope, possibility, and the motivation to keep moving forward into growth and expansion. One of the most powerful prompts in my healing journey was one that invited me to consider my inner landscape and lift up above it to get an eagle's eye view. I had no idea at the time how powerfully God would use this to direct and empower me. Here's a sneak peek into the power of journaling and visualization.

My Visualization Exercise: A Landscape of My Life

As I visualized it, I saw a woman who had reached the midpoint in her life. Behind her were beautiful mountaintops, grassy plains, valleys, and even a few deserts—places she had walked to get to where she was. Markers lined the path, reminders of joys, trials, and the moments she had overcome. I could see how the experiences along the way connected like stepping stones, carrying her to the present moment. She stood frozen on the last stone, staring at the blank canvas of her future. Scattered before her were countless stones leading in different directions. She strained to see which one was "right," afraid to leap onto the wrong path and end up lost. But instead of forcing herself to choose, she sat beside a river flowing nearby and drank deeply from its life-giving water. After some rest, she stood again, refreshed and ready to move. Looking around, she realized she was free to explore. She didn't need permission or a roadmap; she was a grown woman with much to offer and no time to waste.

I saw God smiling down at me and saying, *What are you waiting for? Don't you see the landscape I've laid out for you? I created it for your pleasure! Go enjoy it. I haven't confined or limited you to one specific path—I came to give you freedom. Sweet child, you're so worried about taking the 'right' step that you're just sitting under the shade of the tree by the river when you could jump in a kayak and float downstream. Don't miss the adventure because you're afraid you'll get lost. Whether you choose a kayak, a canoe, a rubber tire, or even ride a horse along the riverbank, I'll guide you. If you wander off course, I'll redirect you.*

As I began to move forward with confidence, I noticed other women traveling through their own landscapes. Some were running, flying kites, and sailing joyfully. Others rode in boats together, while a few sat with their arms around their knees under bridges or inside caves—exhausted, longing for someone to reach down and extend a hand.

I realized I didn't need a new landscape or a change of scenery. I simply needed to start moving and exploring the one I was already in. It didn't feel barren or confining anymore. Looking down from above gave me perspective. All I had to do was put one foot in front of the other. Each step could take me anywhere—the possibilities were endless! The thrill wasn't about skipping to a more desirable place. The journey itself was the reward.

I saw other travelers, too—people I could encourage along the way. I could come alongside them, offer rest if they were tired, listen to their stories, and lead them to the water if they were thirsty. And I could also be content when they walked away, refreshed and ready to carry comfort to someone else. I realized I didn't need crowds of people around me to enjoy my path. I wasn't alone after all.

Walking Hand-in-Hand with the Creator

From this new vantage point, I could see the whole world stretched before me. I could see the paths I had walked, the valleys I had survived, and the mountaintops I had climbed. Ahead of me, the landscape extended further—no longer overwhelming or confusing but full of possibility. I knew there would be dry places, hard places, and hot places ahead. But I also knew that the same God who had carried me through those places before would carry me through them again. I had tasted the fruit that exists beyond those difficult places, and I trusted Him to hold me as I carried what He had entrusted to me. I no longer wanted to escape my landscape. I wanted to stay—fully present, fully engaged. There were no limits. The walls were wide open, and I was free to come and go. Even if I spent days at my computer typing the pages of my story, that story could stretch across the landscape of others' lives and leave an impact.

I am not trapped. I am not stuck. And if I do feel stuck again, I'll pull up a map—reminding myself of the vastness of this world and the truth that God has not set limits on me. His desire is for me to be effective and fruitful, to spread His glory wherever I am. I don't need to get lost in questions of "how" or "what step." As long as I enjoy Him in the landscape I stand on today, He will guide me forward. One day, I'll look back and see where all those steps connected, like arrows radiating across the terrain of my life.

From Reflection to Action

I'm in awe of how God used this exercise I did over 10 years ago during a journaling course led by Amber Lea Starfire to inspire vision and propel me to where I am today. That course was the first of many baby steps I took. While that specific course isn't available anymore, Amber continues to share inspiring journaling prompts and tools for self-reflection on her website, *Writing Through Life*.[51]

GOOD GIRL RX: Take Empowered Action

Clarity doesn't come from waiting; it comes from engagement—moving forward, one small step at a time. Sometimes, all it takes is a pause, a deep breath, and the willingness to shift your weight. *Small steps swing big doors. You've got this; just start leaning into what feels inviting!*

Reflection Questions:

1. What will your next step be? What small action can you take today that moves you toward the life you desire?
2. What is your body and soul feeling drawn to explore more? Where do you feel curious or excited? Follow that feeling.
3. When you get an eagle's-eye view, what do you see? What does the landscape of your life look like from this perspective?

---

51 Starfire, Amber Lea. *Writing Through Life*. www.writingthroughlife.com.

Thank you for taking this journey with me. Your voice matters, and I'd love to hear from you. If you have questions, reflections, or topics you'd love more of just reach out. You can find me at katebartley.com

www.ingramcontent.com/pod-product-compliance
Lightning Source LLC
Chambersburg PA
CBHW020535030426
42337CB00013B/866